O R M L
OXFORD RESPIRATORY MEDICINE LIBRARY

Cystic Fibrosis

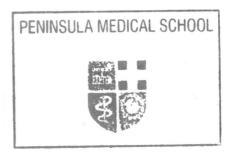

PENINSULA MEDICAL SCHOOL

D0755878

Oxford University Press makes no representation, express or implied, that the drug dosages in this book are correct. Readers must therefore always check the product information and clinical procedures with the most up-to-date published product information and data sheets provided by the manufacturers and the most recent codes of conduct and safety regulations. The authors and the publishers do not accept responsibility or legal liability for any errors in the text or for the misuse or misapplication of material in this work.

▶ Except where otherwise stated, drug doses and recommendations are for the non-pregnant adult who is not breast-feeding.

ORML

OXFORD RESPIRATORY MEDICINE LIBRARY

Cystic Fibrosis

Edited by

Dr Alex Horsley

Senior Fellow,
Manchester Adult Cystic Fibrosis Centre,
University Hospital of South Manchester,
Wythenshawe Hospital
Manchester, UK

Dr Steve Cunningham

Consultant Respiratory Paediatrician and Part Time
Senior Lecturer, Department of Child Life & Health,
Royal Hospital for Sick Children,
Edinburgh, UK

Dr J. Alastair Innes

Consultant Physician and Honorary Reader in
Respiratory Medicine, Scottish Adult CF Service,
Western General Hospital, Edinburgh, UK

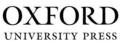

OXFORD
UNIVERSITY PRESS

OXFORD
UNIVERSITY PRESS

Great Clarendon Street, Oxford OX2 6DP

Oxford University Press is a department of the University of Oxford.
It furthers the University's objective of excellence in research, scholarship,
and education by publishing worldwide in

Oxford New York

Auckland Cape Town Dar es Salaam Hong Kong Karachi
Kuala Lumpur Madrid Melbourne Mexico City Nairobi
New Delhi Shanghai Taipei Toronto

With offices in

Argentina Austria Brazil Chile Czech Republic France Greece
Guatemala Hungary Italy Japan Poland Portugal Singapore
South Korea Switzerland Thailand Turkey Ukraine Vietnam

Oxford is a registered trade mark of Oxford University Press
in the UK and in certain other countries

Published in the United States
by Oxford University Press Inc., New York

British Library Cataloguing in Publication Data

Data available

Library of Congress Cataloging in Publication Data

Data available

Typeset by Newgen Imaging Systems (P) Ltd., Chennai, India
Printed in Great Britain
on acid-free paper by
Ashford Colour Press Ltd., Gosport, Hamshire
ISBN 978–0–19–958270–9

10 9 8 7 6 5 4 3 2 1

Whilst every effort has been made to ensure that the contents of this book are as
complete, accurate and-up-to-date as possible at the date of writing, Oxford
University Press is not able to give any guarantee or assurance that such is the case.
Readers are urged to take appropriately qualified medical advice in all cases. The
information in this book is intended to be useful to the general reader, but should
not be used as a means of self-diagnosis or for the prescription of medication.

Contents

Preface

The outlook for patients with Cystic Fibrosis (CF) can be regarded as both a success and an ongoing challenge for modern medicine. On the one hand, life expectancy has improved enormously over the past 3–4 decades, and what was once viewed as an exclusively paediatric disease now affects more adults than children in many Western countries. We now also have a good understanding of the genetic basis of the disease, and some understanding of the patho-physiology. Improved survival has come about through advances in the treatment of pulmonary infections, as well as in the management of the nutritional and metabolic consequences of the disease. On the other hand, the result of this is an increasing treatment burden for the patients and, despite being a single gene disorder, a genetic cure remains elusive.

Pulmonary infections and progressive respiratory failure are the primary causes of mortality and morbidity, and patients are usually cared for by respiratory specialist teams. CF however is a multi-system disease, and the treatment and management of patients with CF necessarily involves many different specialists, from different disciplines of medicine and associated professions. As patients live longer, the importance of managing these other complications becomes more pressing, and it is clear that earlier recognition and treatment of non-respiratory complications will form an important part of future CF care. This book is aimed at all involved in the care of CF patients and we hope that we have succeeded in covering the broad range of problems faced by the both adult and paediatric teams.

Much of the management of patients with CF is based upon what is thought to be best practice, rather than large randomized controlled trials. There is therefore bound to be some variation in practice between different units and countries. Where suggestions have been made, in the absence of unequivocal evidence, they remain just that, and may differ from local policy. We hope however that where guidance has been offered that it will prove useful, even if not identical to local practice.

Alex Horsley
Steve Cunningham
J. Alastair Innes
Edinburgh 2010

Contributors

Eric Alton
Professor of Respiratory Medicine and Gene Therapy, Honorary Consultant Physician, Royal Brompton and Harefield Hospital, Department of Gene Therapy National Heart & Lung Institute Imperial College, London, UK

Sally Connolly
Consultant Paediatrician, Sheffield Children's Hospital, Sheffield, UK

Steve Cunningham
Consultant Respiratory Paediatrician & Part Time Senior Lecturer, Department of Child Life & Health Royal Hospital for Sick Children, Edinburgh, UK

Jane Davies
Reader in Paediatric Respiratory Medicine and Gene Therapy, Honorary Consultant, Royal Brompton and Harefield Hospital, National Heart & Lung Institute Imperial College, London, UK

Gerd Döring
Professor and Head of Cystic Fibrosis Research Group, Institute of Medical Microbiology and Hygiene, University of Tübingen, Tübingen, Germany

Alistair Duff
Consultant Clinical Psychologist & Honorary Senior Lecturer, Head of Psychology Services, Leeds Teaching Hospitals & Leeds University School of Medicine, Leeds, UK

Frank Edenborough
Consultant Respiratory Physician Clinical Lead, Sheffield Adult CF Centre, Northern General Hospital, Sheffield, UK

Andrew J. Fisher
Professor of Respiratory Transplant Medicine & Honorary Consultant Chest Physician, Cardiopulmonary Transplant Unit, Freeman Hospital, Newcastle Upon Tyne, UK

Uta Griesenbach
Reader in Molecular Medicine, National Heart & Lung Institute, Imperial College, London, UK

Charles Haworth
Consultant Respiratory Physician, Adult Cystic Fibrosis Centre and Lung Defence Unit, Papworth Hospital, Cambridge, UK

Alex Horsley
Senior Fellow, Manchester Adult Cystic Fibrosis Centre, University Hospital of South Manchester, Wythenshawe Hospital, Manchester, UK

J. Alastair Innes
Consultant Physician and Honorary Reader in Respiratory Medicine, Scottish Adult CF Service, Western General Hospital, Edinburgh, UK

CONTRIBUTORS

Antoinette Moran
Division Chief & Professor of
Paediatric Endocrinology,
University of Minnesota,
Minneapolis, USA

Stephen M.P. O'Riordan
Clinician Researcher in Diabetes,
Endocrinology and CFRD,
The Institute of Child Health &
Great Ormond Street Hospital,
London, UK

Helen Oxley
Consultant Clinical Psychologist,
Manchester Adult CF Centre,
Wythenshawe Hospital
Manchester, UK

Laura Tanner
Specialist Registrar in Respiratory
Medicine,
Cardiopulmonary Transplant Unit,
Freeman Hospital,
Newcastle Upon Tyne, UK

Christopher Taylor
Professor of Paediatric
Gastroenterology,
Academic Unit of Child Health,
University of Sheffield,
Sheffield, UK

Dieter Worlitzsch
Senior Physician & Specialist for
Hygiene and Environmental
Medicine,
Institute of Hygiene, University
Hospital of Halle,
Halle, Germany

In addition, the editors gratefully
acknowledge the input of:

Emma Williamson
Consultant Microbiologist,
New Royal Infirmary,
Edinburgh, UK

Sarah Ridley
Senior Respiratory
Physiotherapist,
Scottish Adult CF Service,
Western General Hospital,
Edinburgh, UK

Abbreviations

AAV	adeno-associated virus
ABC	ATP-binding cassette
ABPA	allergic bronchopulmonary aspergillosis
ACBT	active cycle of breathing technique
AD	autogenic drainage
ADA	American Diabetes Association
BCC	*Burkholderia cepacia* complex bacteria
BG	blood glucose
BMD	bone mineral density
BMI	body mass index
BOS	bronchiolitis obliterans syndrome
BPFAS	Behavioral Pediatric Feeding Assessment Scale
CBAVD	congenital bilateral absence of the vas deferens
CBT	cognitive behaviour therapy
CDI	Children's Depression Inventory
CF	cystic fibrosis
CFRD	CF related diabetes
CFRD FH+	diabetes with fasting hyperglycemia
CFRD FH-	diabetes without fasting hyperglycemia
CFTR	cystic fibrosis transmembrane conductance regulator
CFQ	Cystic Fibrosis Questionnaire
CFQ-UK	CF Questionnaire
CGM	continuous glucose monitoring
CMV	cytomegalovirus
CT	computed tomography
DIOS	distal ileal obstruction syndrome
DXA	dual energy x-ray absorptiometry
ENaC	transepithelial sodium channel
ERCF	European Epidemiologic Registry of Cystic Fibrosis
GORD	gastro-oesophageal reflux disease
GTA	gene transfer agents
HADS	Hospital Anxiety and Depression Scale

HCG	human chorionic gonadotrophin
HIVT	home intravenous antibiotic treatment
HRCT	high-resolution computed tomography
HRQoL	health-related quality of life
IAPP	islet amyloid polypeptide
IBAT	ileal bile acid transporter
ICSI	intracytoplasmic sperm injection
IGT	impaired glucose tolerance
IRT	immune reactive trypsin
ISPAD	International Society of Pediatric Adolescent Diabetes
IUD	intrauterine devices
IVF	in vitro fertilization techniques
MRSA	methicillin resistant *Staphylococcus aureus*
NG	nasogastric
NGT	normal glucose tolerance
NIV	non-invasive positive pressure ventilation
NTM	non-tuberculous mycobacteria
OGTT	oral glucose tolerance testing
OPEP	oscillating positive expiratory pressure
PCP	*Pneumocystis jirovecci*
PCR	polymerase chain reaction
PEG	percutaneous endoscopic gastrostomy
PEP	positive expiratory pressure
PERT	pancreatic enzyme replacement therapy
PESA	percutaneous epididymal sperm aspiration
PGD	pre-implantation genetic diagnosis
PI	pancreatic insufficiency
PICC	peripherally inserted central catheters
PTLD	post transplant lymphoproliferative disorder
PsA	*Pseudomonas aeruginosa*
PVL	Panton-Valentine leukocidin
QoL	quality of life
RDR	recommended daily requirements
SACS	Spence Children's Anxiety Scales
TB	tuberculosis

TESA	testicular sperm aspiration
TESE	testicular sperm extraction
TIPPS	transjugular intra-hepatic portosystemic shunting
TIVAD	totally indwelling venous access device
TLC	total lung capacity
WHO	World Health Organization

Chapter 1

Genetics and pathophysiology

Alex Horsley

'The child will soon die whose forehead tastes salty when kissed'
(Almanac of Children's Songs and Games,
Switzerland 1857)

Key points

- Cystic fibrosis (CF) is the most common autosomal recessive disease in Caucasians associated with early death
- Unaffected carrier frequency is 1:25
- Phe508del is the most common of over 1,500 mutations.
- The gene encodes a transmembrane chloride conductance channel, the CFTR, which regulates chloride ion and water movements across the cell membrane
- CFTR is expressed throughout the body, and CF disease affects multiple systems, including major effects on the lung, pancreas and gastrointestinal systems
- Pulmonary disease is the most important cause of death and disability, resulting from chronic progressive suppurative lung disease
- Over-activation of the sodium (ENaC) channel in the lungs, caused by loss of CFTR-inhibition, results in dehydration of the airway surface fluid layer and consequent poor mucociliary clearance
- Retained secretions encourage bacterial adherence, chronic neutrophillic infection, and a vicious cycle of infection, inflammation and tissue destruction.

1.1 Introduction

Cystic fibrosis (CF) is a complex multisystem disease, caused by defects in a single gene. Pulmonary manifestations are responsible for most of the morbidity and mortality, and the hallmark of the condition is progressive and irreversible bronchiectasis and respiratory failure. However, the condition also has effects on gastrointestinal function, nutrition, endocrine, metabolic, and reproductive systems.

1.2 Genetics

Cystic fibrosis is the most common life-shortening genetic disorder of Caucasians. The faulty gene, on the long arm of chromosome 7, was identified in 1989, and encodes an epithelial ion channel known as the cystic fibrosis transmembrane conductance regulator (CFTR). Carriers of a single faulty gene are asymptomatic and CF is caused by co-inheritance of two disease-causing mutant alleles of the CFTR gene, one from each parent (Figure 1.1). The condition has a carrier frequency of 1:25 in those of European descent and affects 1 in 2500 live births in the UK and Western Europe. This high incidence may be explained by a possible protective effect in CF carriers, against gastrointestinal infections such typhoid or cholera.

1.2.1 CFTR Mutations

Over 1,500 CFTR mutations have been described, but the most common mutation is a deletion of three base pairs (CTT) encoding phenylalanine at position 508, known as Phe508del (Phe = phenylalanine, del = deletion). This was previously known as ΔF508 (Δ = 'delta', or deletion, and F=phenylalanine). This is largely responsible

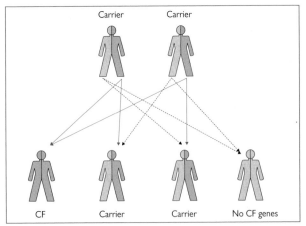

Figure 1.1 Inheritance of CF. Each parent carries a single copy of a defective CF gene (illustrated as blue shading), but because they have one normal copy they are asymptomatic. There is a 1:4 chance of producing a CF child, and half of children will also be carriers.

for the high incidence of CF in the Caucasian population, where it accounts for over two thirds of CF mutations. Many patients will be compound heterozygotes, containing one copy of the Phe508del gene and one other mutation.

CF mutations vary in how they affect CFTR function. Those mutations leaving little functioning CFTR tend to have the most significant clinical effect, whereas those mutations leaving some residual CFTR function may exhibit milder disease. Milder mutations in compound heterozygotes have a dominant effect (i.e. a severe and a mild mutation combined will usually have mild disease).

Class of mutation

CF mutations are grouped into six classes depending on their effect on gene expression and CFTR function (see Figure 1.2).

- Class I: Transcription errors resulting in unstable, truncated or no protein expression
- Class II: Defective protein maturation and trafficking. Phe508del is an example of this sort of mutation
- Class III: Impaired chloride channel activity. These mutations primarily affect the two nucleotide binding domains (NBD), see Figure 1.4.
- Class IV: Defective channel gating and reduced chloride conductance
- Class V: Splicing abnormalities resulting in reduced amounts of functional protein
- Class VI: Accelerated turnover.

Relationship between genotype and phenotype

Clinical severity is broadly related to the amount of residual CFTR activity. At one end of the spectrum (class I and II), little or no CFTR activity usually gives rise to severe lung disease. With increasing levels of residual CFTR function (class III, IV, V), pancreatic sufficiency is maintained, which has important prognostic implications. For instance, the presence of the class IV mutation R117H is reliably associated with pancreatic sufficiency. Just under 5% of the healthy CFTR mRNA levels appear to be sufficient to prevent the development of severe lung disease. Class V mutations may be associated with particularly mild phenotypes (e.g. congenital bilateral absence of vas deferens, with no other clinical manifestations of CF).

A list of common mutations, and their clinical effects, is given in Table 1.1. There are distinct differences in allele frequencies between the Caucasian population, and those of different ethnic background, which has implications for screening.

Modifiers of CF phenotype

Even amongst patients with the same genotype however, there is considerable variability in disease progression. The reasons for this are multi-factorial, and include social and environmental factors, such

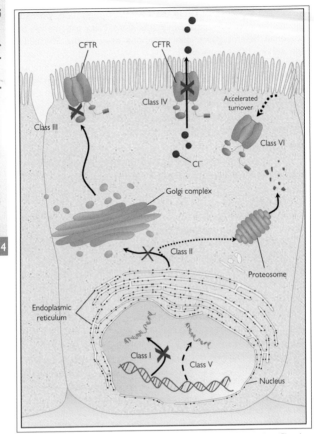

Figure 1.2 Classes of CFTR mutation and their effect on gene expression. Class I mutation – transcription errors; Class II – defective protein maturation and trafficking; Class III – impaired chloride channel activity; Class IV – defective channel gating; Class V – splicing abnormalities; Class VI – accelerated turnover. The first two of these are associated with particularly diminished or absent CFTR activity and often with more severe clinical phenotypes. Adapted from Rowe et al. (2005).

as access to specialist healthcare and compliance with treatment regimens (Figure 1.3). Modifier genes are also believed to play an important role in this individual disease variability. Modifier genes are polymorphisms that provide genetic variation in all individuals (i.e. what kind of cytokine response we have to a standard stimulus etc), but which in CF may have important implications for the response to infection and inflammation.

Table 1.1 Frequency of common CFTR mutations in the UK

Mutation	Class	Frequency (%)		Notes
		Caucasian	Asian*	
Phe508del	II	74.1	29.5	
G551D	III	3.37	12.8	Associated with lower frequency of meconium ileus and later age of PI
G542X	I	1.85	25.6	Associated with PI
R117H	IV	1.25	0	Mild mutation, associated with preserved pancreatic function, minimal or no respiratory symptoms and CBAVD
621+1G→T	I	1.27	6.4	
Y569D	III	0.15	9.62	Common in UK Pakistani popn.
L218X	I	0.06	3.85	
1161delC	I	0.07	3.85	
R1162X	I	0.09	1.92	Associated with PI, but mild-moderate lung disease
R709X	I	0.04	1.28	Associated with pancreatic sufficiency
3849+10kb→T	V	0.12	1.92	

*Asian refers to those of Pakistani, Indian, Bangladeshi and other Asian descent.
CBAVD: Congenital bilateral absence of the vas deferens (male infertility).
PI: Pancreatic insufficiency.
Adapted from McCormick et al. (2002).

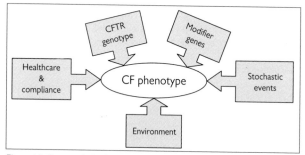

Figure 1.3 Factors which influence the severity of CF lung disease. Stochastic events are random, unpredictable events.

Table 1.2 Proposed CF modifier genes		
Category	Effect	Examples
Ion & water transport	Ion channels	ENaC Alternative Cl⁻ and K⁺ channels
	Ion channel activation	β_2-AR
Immunity and airway defence	Antigen presentation	HLA locus
	Innate defences	Mannose-Binding Lectin 2 Nitric oxide synthases
	Inflammation cascade (cytokines)	TNFα IL-8 IL-10
	Neutrophil regulation	IFRD1
	Mucins	MUC5A
Lung injury and repair	Proteases and anti-proteases	Neutrophil elastase, α_1-antitrypsin α_1-antichymotrypsin
	Oxidants/anti-oxidants	Glutathione S-transferase (also linked to liver disease)
	Tissue growth factors	TGF-β
	Toxic cell injury	Acid sphingomyelinase
Intra-cellular processing of CFTR		Heat shock proteins (hsp70)

A number of modifier genes have been identified that may affect the severity of the clinical phenotype in a variety of ways. These include proteins that CFTR interacts with directly, such as other ion channels in the epithelial membrane, as well genes that act indirectly on the CF phenotype, such as those related to antigen processing and host defence. A list of possible modifier genes is given in Table 1.2. Most of these remain putative, and often based upon relatively small studies. Of the proposed genes, the most convincing evidence for modifier effects exists for TGF-β (a cytokine involved in cell proliferation and differentiation and the regulation of fibrosis) and Mannose-Binding Lectin (MBL) 2 (a component of the innate immune system that binds micro-organisms and promotes phagocytosis).

1.3 Cystic fibrosis transmembrane regulator (CFTR)

1.3.1 Structure and function of CFTR

The protein encoded by the CFTR gene comprises 1,480 amino acids. CFTR is a member of a class of proteins termed the ATP-binding cassette (ABC). The protein spans cell membranes at

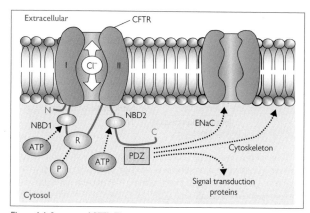

Figure 1.4 Structure of CFTR. The protein is expressed in apical cell membranes where it functions as a chloride channel. The channel is made up of two membrane spanning domains (I and II), each consisting of 6 membrane spanning alpha helices. Two nucleotide binding domains (NBD1 and NBD2) mediate ATP hydrolysis, and it is on one of these (NBD1) that the most common CFTR mutation (Phe508del) occurs. Phosphorylation of the R domain permits a conformational change and opening of the channel. CFTR binds a seperate PDZ domain at its C terminus, through which it interacts with an array of different cellular proteins, including cytoskeleton, cell signaling mechanisms, and other ion channels - in particular the epithelial sodium channel ENaC.

two adjacent points to form a central channel (Figure 1.4). CFTR protein also has two nucleotide binding domains (NBD 1 & 2), which are capable of opening and closing the channel by hydrolysis of ATP. CFTR functions as a channel for chloride and (to a lesser extent) bicarbonate ions, and is flow regulated by protein kinase A.

CFTR in the sweat glands is normally responsible for chloride, and hence sodium, reabsorption. It is the failure of this mechanism in CF that leads to excessive excretion of salt, and the salty taste described in the Swiss nursery rhyme quoted at the start of the chapter. This also forms the basis of the sweat test for diagnosis of CF (see Chapter 2).

The Phe508del mutation occurs on NBD1 and prevents normal folding into the appropriate tertiary structure, resulting in cellular retention and degradation (a class II mutation, see Figure 1.2).

1.3.2 Interaction with other proteins

CFTR forms part of a multi-protein assembly in the apical plasma membrane, and is involved in the regulation of a number of cellular processes. In particular it acts to down-regulate the activity of the transepithelial sodium channel (ENaC) in the apical epithelial membrane, an interaction with important consequences for the effects in the lung. In addition to this, it also interacts with calcium-activated chloride channels, potassium channels, sodium-bicarbonate transporters and aquaporin water channels. Variability in the function of these other proteins are potential modifiers of the CF phenotype. CFTR is also able to form dimers in the plasma membrane, which may act to increase channel activity and/or reduce endocytic retrieval of CFTR from the membrane.

1.4 Pathophysiology

CFTR is expressed in epithelia throughout the body, and affects exocrine (secretory) function in a number of organs, including the lung, liver, gut, pancreas and sweat glands. Most of the epithelial sites of expression correspond well with the known clinical effects of CF (Figure 1.5). The extra-pulmonary effects of CF will be described in the individual chapters dealing with these organs. The pulmonary manifestations however are the most important in terms of the burden of disease and survival

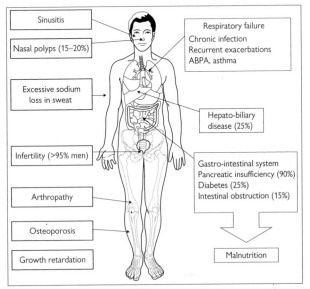

Figure 1.5 Clinical consequences of CF. Percentages in brackets represent the approximate percentages of CF patients affected in this way.

1.4.1 Lung disease in cystic fibrosis

In the lung, CFTR is detectable on the apical membrane of ciliated cells within the gland ducts and in the superficial epithelium of healthy individuals. In CF, the submucosal glands and distal airways are obstructed by thick tenacious secretions, resulting in a failure of normal mucociliary clearance and defective airway defence mechanisms against bacterial infection.

Low volume hypothesis

The most widely accepted explanation for the clinical effects of CFTR deficiency in the lung is known as the low volume hypothesis (see Figure 1.6). This proposes that, since CFTR normally functions

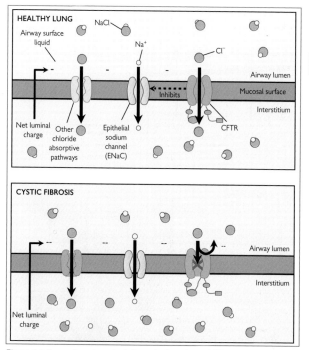

Figure 1.6 Low volume hypothesis for pathophysiology of CF in airway epithelium. In the normal airway (top), CFTR absorbs chloride ions (Cl⁻), and regulates absorption of sodium (Na⁺) through ENaC channels. In CF, inhibition of ENaC is abolished, leading to hyper-absorption of Na⁺. Cl⁻ follows through alternative Cl⁻ channels, and water follows, leading to shrinkage of the airway surface liquid and hyperpolarisation of the epithelial surface (increased negative charge).

to down-regulate ENaC, loss of CFTR function leads to over-activity of ENaC. Excessive Na^+ is therefore absorbed, and Cl^- follows through non-CFTR Cl^- channels. Mouse models with defective CFTR do not exhibit the classic pulmonary features of CF, whereas a mouse model with excessive ENaC activity has a lung phenotype similar to that of human CF. This leads to net absorption of ions and fluid, with consequent shrinking of the pericilliary layer of airway surface liquid, dehydration of mucous secretions and collapse of epithelial cilia (Figure 1.7). The effects on the mucus layer and the cilia are crucial in the development of CF lung disease. In health, the mucus layer is a gel consisting of around 1% salt, 1% high molecular weight

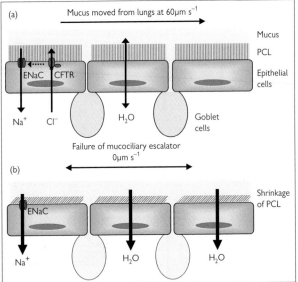

Figure 1.7 Proposed mechanism for the development of chronic airway infection in CF, after Boucher (2007). In normal airways (a), hydration is controlled by Na^+ absorption (inhibited by CTFR) & Cl^- secretion. In CF (b), the absence of CFTR leads to unregulated Na^+ absorption and associated dehydration of the periciliary layer (PCL) and mucus. Mucus becomes adherent in plaques which allow bacterial colonisation (c), causing mucus hypersecretion and encouraged by a hypoxic gradient across the plaque. The resulting inflammatory response (d) leads to a vicious cycle of inflammation, mucus secretion and retention, and ultimately airway destruction. Reprinted, with permission, from the *Annual Review of Medicine*, Volume 58, © 2007 by Annual Reviews (www.annualreviews.org).

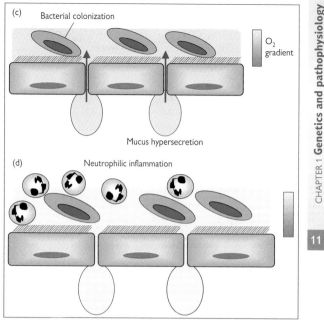

Figure 1.7 *Continued*

secreted mucins and 98% water. At its inner surface, between the mucus layer and the epithelial cell membrane, lies a thin pericilliary liquid layer. This layer provides a low viscosity solution in which the cilia can beat rapidly. It also prevents adhesion of the mucus to the epithelial surface, thereby lubricating the movement of mucus during cough clearance. Healthy airway epithelia in culture maintain an airway surface liquid layer depth of 7μm, but CF airway epithelia continue to absorb the surface liquid and the cilia collapse onto the cell surface.

Effects on mucus clearance

Unregulated absorption of ions and water across the CF airway epithelium causes shrinkage of the pericilliary layer (PCL) of surface liquid and dehydration of the overlying mucus layer (Figure 1.7). Shrinkage of the PCL impairs the action of the cilia and brings an increasingly adhesive mucus layer into contact with the epithelium. The disruption of mucociliary clearance leads to mucus plugging, which causes airway obstruction and promotes bacterial infection.

Vicious cycle of infection and inflammation

The exact process by which infection occurs is unclear, but may comprise inhaled bacteria that are not cleared efficiently, or the initial infection may follow an insult to the lung such as viral infection or aspiration. Whatever the initiating event, lungs of CF patients often become colonized early in the course of the disease with bacteria such as Staphylococci or *H. influenzae*. These infections become persistent in the first few years of life and there is a florid inflammatory response that leads to neutrophil recruitment and activation. This in turn stimulates hypersecretion of mucin. Bacterial products and cellular debris accumulate, along with polymeric DNA (from bacteria and neutrophils) which makes the mucus more viscous and even harder to expel. The persisting neutrophil-dominated inflammatory response leads to release of neutrophil proteases, such as elastase and matrix metallo-proteinases. These cause proteolysis and chondrolysis of airway support tissue, with consequent airway dilatation and bronchiectasis. The CF airways fill up with purulent secretions and a vicious cycle of infection, inflammation and progressive endobronchial destruction is established (Figure 1.8).

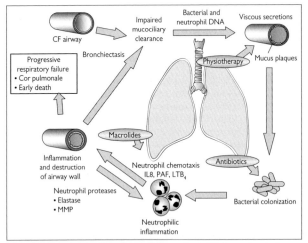

Figure 1.8 Vicious cycle of infection and inflammation in CF airways. Impaired mucociliary clearance in CF leads to retention of mucus, allowing bacterial colonization and subsequent neutrophillic inflammation. This results in mucosal and airway wall damage, progressing to bronchiectasis and ultimately to respiratory failure. Therapeutic interventions are shown in blue ovals, with the proposed site of action indicated.

1.4.2 Clinical course

The manifestations of CF lung disease are highly variable in onset and intensity. The clinical course is typically punctuated by periods of exacerbation, when bacterial infection gains the upper hand over host defence. At these times there is usually deterioration in lung function, and associated symptoms of infection (see Chapter 5). Some organisms, particularly *Pseudomonas aeruginosa* and *Burkholderia cepacia* (see Chapter 3), are associated with greater inflammation.

Chronic Pseudomonas infection

Pseudomonas aeruginosa is an important opportunistic infection in CF with important clinical consequences, and becomes established in the majority of patients by their late teens (see Chapter 3). It exists in two forms; a non-mucoid form and a mucoid form that, once established, is resistant to eradication. The formation of mucoid *Pseudomonas* biofilms appears to be encouraged by the thickened mucus in the CF airways. Mucus limits bacterial motility and diffusion of excreted proteins and the resulting high bacterial densities are detected by the bacteria's quorum-sensing mechanisms, which triggers a phenotypic change to biofilm forms. In addition, the thick mucus layer and the increased oxygen consumption of the epithelial cells lead to an oxygen gradient across the mucus, with particularly hypoxic areas in mucus plugs. This hypoxic environment favours the growth of *Pseudomonas* and switching to biofilm formation (Figure 1.7).

1.4.3 CFTR and the immune system

Impaired mucociliary clearance may not be the only significant process occurring in the CF lung however. Other diseases are also associated with failure of mucociliary clearance, in particular primary ciliary dyskinesia, which has bronchiectasis as a common clinical feature, but generally has a far greater life expectancy than is seen in CF.

In patients with CF, a number of studies of infant bronchoalveolar lavage (BAL) fluid have found evidence of airway inflammation without concurrent lower airway infection. It may be that defective CFTR leads to dysregulation of the host defences in other, more complex ways.

The innate defences of the airways consist of three main components, and there is evidence for deficiency in all three of these in CF (Figure 1.9). Impairment of the physical defence provided by the mucociliary escalator is described above, and is certainly a major component of the lung pathophysiology in CF. There may also be impairment in the humoral defences, including defensins, antioxidants such as glutathione S transferase, and surfactant proteins.

Lastly, there is increasing evidence for impairments in cell mediated immunity. CFTR is involved in lysosomal acidification via the counter-effect of Cl⁻ on H⁺ accumulation, and this may be deficient in CF. CF neutrophils also appear to have an exaggerated response to inflammatory stimuli, associated with a reduced ability to phagocytose and clear bacteria. It is likely that a combination of these different mechanisms is responsible for the sustained inflammation that is the hallmark of CF pulmonary disease.

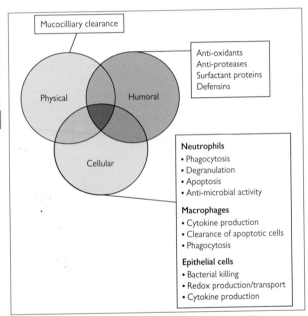

Figure 1.9 Effects of CF on innate immune system. Lung disease in CF is a consequence not purely of dysfunctional mucociliary clearance but also impairments in humoral and cellular immunity. The final phenotype is a consequence of the interaction between all of these factors.

References

McCormick J., Green M.W., Mehta G., Culross F., Mehta A. (2002) Demographics of the UK cystic fibrosis population: implications for screening. *Eur. J. Hum. Genet.* **10**: 583–90.

Rowe S.M., Miller S., Sorscher E.J. (2005) Cystic fibrosis. *N. Engl. J. Med.* **352**: 1992–2001.

Guggino W.B., Stanton B.A. (2006) New insights into cystic fibrosis: molecular switches that regulate CFTR. *Nat. Rev. Mol. Cell Biol.* **7**: 426–36.

Boucher R.C. (2007) Airway surface dehydration in cystic fibrosis: pathogenesis and therapy. *Annu. Rev. Med.* **58**: 157–70.

Doring G., Gulbins E. (2009) Cystic fibrosis and innate immunity: how chloride channels provoke lung disease. *Cellular Microbiology* **11**: 208–16.

Collaco J.M., Cutting G.R. (2008) Update on gene modifiers in cystic fibrosis. *Curr. Opin. Pulm. Med.* **14**: 559–66.

Chapter 2

Diagnosis and process of care

Steve Cunningham

Key points

- Diagnosis is most common in those with recurrent respiratory infection and poor weight gain in the first year of life
- Those not diagnosed as newborns may present later in life with more subtle, but troublesome, respiratory infection
- CF is a clinical diagnosis, supported by an abnormal sweat chloride level on sweat testing
- Genetic analysis may help confirm a diagnosis of CF, but the very large number of mutations now identified make some genotype/phenotype relationships difficult to predict
- Newborn screening programmes generally test for raised immune reactive trypsin (IRT) on blood taken within the first week of life, with a subsequent test for CF gene mutations if IRT is elevated
- Patients with CF require regular review by health professionals trained in CF care
- Patients with CF may inadvertently share respiratory organisms and consideration should be given as how to minimize this risk during hospital contact.
- Annual review is an important event in the care of patients with CF, enabling a multidisciplinary perspective on the rate of disease progression and plans made to slow this decline
- Transition to adult services should begin in early teens, actively involve patients and parents, and provide plenty of opportunity for transfer of information across teams.

2.1 Presentation

Cystic fibrosis classically presents with failure to thrive and recurrent respiratory infection in the first few months of life. Clinical features at diagnosis, and timing of presentation, depend to a significant extent on patient genotype. The understanding of genotype/phenotype relationships is still evolving, but broadly divides into those with pancreatic sufficiency (c15%) and insufficiency (c85%).

2.1.1 Newborn

Meconium ileus is an obstruction of the terminal ileum with inspissated meconium (see Chapter 6). It occurs in the first few days of life, and often requires surgery to remove both the obstruction and any associated necrotic intestine.

Meconium ileus is a presenting feature in up to around 20% of infants with CF. 80% of cases of meconium ileus occur in patients subsequently diagnosed with CF.

Meconium ileus does not occur more frequently in any particular CF genotype.

2.1.2 Young children

Patients presenting in the first five years of life tend to be pancreatic insufficient. Malapsorption makes adequate weight gain difficult (unless weight is maintained by a voracious appetite and frequent stooling). Failure to thrive in such individuals is usually associated with recurrent respiratory infection. In many countries, with the advent of newborn screening (discussed later), such a presentation is now uncommon and often more subtle presentations take place. In areas without newborn screening a high level of suspicion should prompt sweat testing in any infant with poor growth and/or recurrent respiratory symptoms.

2.1.3 Older children and young adults

Presentation in older children and young adults tend to occur in those with pancreatic sufficiency, so called 'milder' genotypes, or in those where classical symptoms and signs have not been appreciated by parents or clinical staff. Pancreatic sufficient genotypes may present with recurrent respiratory infection (sometimes unusual community acquired respiratory infections, particularly atypical mycobacteria), productive cough and bronchiectasis, chronic pancreatitis, diabetes, or infertility in males.

'Asthma' that is poorly responsive to treatment and/or associated with sputum production should raise suspicion of CF. A high index of suspicion should also be maintained for presumed diagnoses (e.g. tuberculosis with bronchiectasis) that may in fact be CF.

2.1.4 **Third decade onward**

Diagnosis in the third decade and older often follows the investigation of grumbling respiratory infections (particularly with unusual organisms and associated finger clubbing), chronic pancreatitis, diabetes, gallstones, recurrent nasal polyps or couple infertility treatment (with male infertility from CABVD). A small proportion present with liver disease (varices, splenomegaly) without obvious signs in the chest.

Some patients have been diagnosed following the diagnosis of their (or a relative's) child identified by newborn screening.

2.2 **Diagnosis**

2.2.1 **CF is a clinical diagnosis**

Recurrent respiratory infection, with the associated development of bronchiectasis and progressive decline in respiratory function, associated with malabsorption, diabetes, liver disease, pancreatitis, nasal polyps, sinusitis and male infertility, is consistent with the diagnosis. A positive sweat test and/or two functional mutations of the CF gene confirm the diagnosis. The sweat test is abnormal in nearly all cases, though results may fall within a normal/borderline range in pancreatic sufficient genotypes throughout life, but particularly in the first year of life.

2.2.2 **CFTR genetic variants**

The CF gene has multiple (>1500) possible mutations, some of which are not associated with clinical CF disease. The function of the gene mutation (see Chapter 1) may be sufficient for infants to be highlighted by newborn screening programmes (with raised immunoreactive trypsin and rare gene mutations identified on extended gene testing), but without known clinical consequences. The future health of such infants is unknown, and they should not be regarded as having CF (as it is a clinical, not genetic diagnosis), but should be medically monitored to identify any early signs of CFTR dysfunction. Such infants have been called 'pre-CF', suggesting that CF will occur one day, but may be better termed CFTR gene variants, given the social and financial implications of a diagnosis of CF.

2.2.3 **Sweat test**

The sweat test remains the gold standard for confirmation of the clinical diagnosis (see Table 2.1 and Figure 2.1). The salt content of sweat in CF is higher than non-CF individuals, because of the failure of chloride and sodium reabsorption in sweat ducts with deficient CFTR. Parents of young infants with CF not infrequently have noted that their child 'tastes' salty when kissing them. The sweat test is a

Box 2.1 Sweat test methods

Gibson & Cooke (1959) (see Figure 2.1)

- Replaced previous method of placing the patient in plastic bags filled with hot water bottles
- Topical pilocarpine (a parasympathetic stimulant) induces sweat production by iontophoresis (transdermal delivery, enhanced by application of a small electric charge) on arm or back
- Sweat is collected on a pad (gauze or filter paper)
- If sufficient weight of sweat is collected (>75mg in 30 minutes), sweat sodium and chloride will be measured
- Needs experienced technician (>10 per year) and quality control.

Macroduct System

- Similar pilocarpine iontophoresis to Gibson and Cooke
- Collects sweat into a small coil (minimum >15µL in 30 minutes)
- Gibson and Cooke preferred over macroduct.

Conductance

- Measurement of sweat conductivity
- May be used for screening
- Not recommended for diagnostic purposes, and positive tests (Cl⁻>50mmol/l) should be referred for Gibson & Cooke testing.

Table 2.1 Sweat chloride levels

<40mmol/l

- Generally not considered consistent with a diagnosis of CF (though it does happen in some rare cases).

40–60 mmol/l

- Considered 'borderline' i.e. requires further evaluation and may be associated with pancreatic sufficient disease or may develop into clinical CF over time.

>60 mmol/l

- Consistent with a diagnosis of CF.

test to induce and collect sweat, in which sodium, chloride and/or conductance can be measured. Infants generally are 6 weeks of age before they can reliably produce satisfactory sweat volumes to be tested, though testing may be possible once an infant is 48 hours old.

2.2.4 Interpretation of sweat test

Sweat chloride is more reliable than sweat sodium for diagnostic purposes and is considered a better discriminator for use in a reference range (see Table 2.1). An abnormal result should always be confirmed with a second test. A normal result in someone with a strong clinical suspicion of CF should also be repeated. Sweat chloride levels increase with age: lower levels may be considered suspicious in infancy.

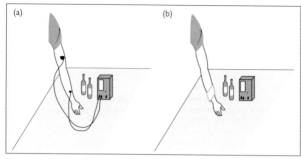

Figure 2.1 Sweat testing. (a) 5 minutes iontoelectrophoresis. Pilocarpine is introduced into the skin by application of a small electric charge. (b) This is followed by 20–30 minutes of sweat collection onto pad or duct collecting system

2.2.5 Interference with sweat test

Contamination is a common cause of interference with the test. Measurement of sweat electrolytes by inexperienced staff leads to more frequent sampling errors, both positive and negative.

Conditions that affect body sodium or water concentration (i.e. malnutrition, nephrogenic diabetes insipidus) or control (i.e. mineralocorticoids) may be associated with anomalous sweat test results.

2.3 Screening for CF

Screening methodologies have predominantly focussed on identifying individuals with severe functional loss of CFTR likely to have clinical CF in early life, though some screening methodologies inadvertently identify individuals with milder degrees of function, where the clinical course is less clear.

2.3.1 Newborn screening

Newborn screening for CF began to develop in earnest in the early 1980's with the recognition that residual exocrine pancreatic function could be assessed by the measurement of immunoreactive trypsin (IRT) on a blood spot from the newborn infant. The IRT continues to be used in most newborn screening programmes for CF as a screening test before the same sample is subsequently assessed for CF gene mutations.

There are many variations to newborn screening schedules, but typically a blood spot from a newborn infant (usually sampled on day 2–6) will be tested for IRT. Infants with an IRT above a declared population cut off (usually ≥99.0% of population IRT), will subsequently have the blood spot screened for a range of CF gene mutations (from

1–31) specific to the mutations most prevalent in the local population. If two CF mutations are identified a diagnosis of CF is made and the family contacted.

If only one CF gene mutation is identified at initial screening some screening programmes may subsequently recall infants for a further IRT measurement at one month. If the second IRT is high (usually ≥99.9% of population IRT), infants are referred for sweat testing and possible further genetic testing. Such infants may be identified not to have CF (false positives), to have CF gene outside the initial genetic test panel (particularly from minority ethic groups), or a rare genotype with an unclear prognosis ('CFTR gene variants').

Newborn screening outcomes

Approximately 20% of infants with CF will be identified following a diagnosis of meconium ileus at birth. Newborn screening programmes may identify up to 80% of the remaining CF population. The health benefits of newborn screening programmes for CF have been less readily demonstrated than many would have hoped. There are improvements in the nutritional status of infants, which continue through childhood to five years of age, but are less distinct thereafter. More ambiguous is the benefit to pulmonary status which remains unproven. The psychological benefit to parents of an early diagnosis must be balanced by the intrusion of a life limiting diagnosis during early bonding.

Clinicians should make themselves aware of the date of introduction of newborn screening in their area, and the likely increased probability of CF diagnosis in those with recurrent respiratory symptoms who were born before screening was introduced.

2.3.2 **Pregnancy associated screening**

Antenatal screening for CF can be population based on a pre-conceptual or antenatal basis, or offered to a targeted population with a family history of CF.

Pre-conception screening

This has not been largely adopted because uptake is generally poor. Many couples either have not heard of CF or consider it relatively uncommon or of limited relevance to them pre-conceptually. Uptake is generally <40% and is not considered cost effective.

Antenatal screening

Antenatal screening is considered to fulfil classic WHO criteria for use of a population screening test. The only routine regional use of antenatal screening was in Edinburgh (UK) from 1991–2003, and was associated with a 65% reduction in diagnosis of CF in the local population. The programme ceased with the introduction of newborn screening.

Box 2.2 Newborn screening methodology dilemmas

The number of infants identified by screening, and the number of false positive and false negatives, will be determined by variations in:

Where to place the population IRT cut off percentage
- A higher percentage improves specificity but reduces sensitivity of test.

What to do with heterozygous single CF genetic results
- The sensitivity of the genetic panel to identify infants with disease in the local population will depend on the size of the panel and the multicultural make up of the local population.

Whether to recall for repeat IRT
- Recalling reduces false positives (from sweat testing all raised IRT/single mutation at first round), but has significant number of false negatives with associated parental anxiety.

What to do with two raised IRT
- Sweat testing may fail to identify an infant with a mild CF mutation. As a consequence it is not possible to definitively confirm to parents that their infant does not have CF.
- Extended genetic testing may identify homozygote mutations for CFTR, though the phenotype of rare mutations are often poorly described.

Pregnancy screening in those with a family history

Couples who have a family history of CF may wish to identify the risk of having a child with CF by pre-conceptual screening of both partners. Where a CF mutation is identified in both partners, there will be a 1 in 4 risk of a pregnancy being affected by CF (see Figure 1.1). Couples with a 1 in 4 risk may opt to continue with the accepted risk, to undergo genetic screening of embryos by pre-implantation diagnosis, or to have chorionic villous genetic screening of the foetus at 11–12 weeks gestation with a view to termination of an affected foetus (see Chapter 11).

2.4 Practical organisation of care

2.4.1 Out-patient

Regular review of patients with CF by professionals with an expert knowledge of the disease improves health outcomes. Out-patient review is typically once per month for young children or those with advanced disease, reducing to a minimum of 3 monthly in those who are generally well.

Health professionals who should contribute to the regular review are:
- Medical clinician with an expert knowledge of CF
- Clinical nurse specialist for CF
- Respiratory physiotherapist
- Specialist dietitian
- Respiratory physiologist
- Psychologist
- Social worker

Nosocomial cross infection of patients with CF may occur during hospital contact. In some reports, multiresistant strains of typical CF respiratory organisms have become endemic across clinic populations, prompting a reappraisal of clinic models in recent years (see Box 2.3).

2.4.2 Routine clinic review

Signs and symptoms in CF are often subtle early in the disease. Recognition requires regular close monitoring by those experienced in CF care. See Box 2.4 for a summary of important points to be considered at clinic review.

Box 2.3 Types of clinic model

Cepacia only segregation
Segregate only patients colonized with *B. cepacia* (see Chapter 3)—hold separate clinic days for *B. cepacia* patients. All other patients attend together on another day.

Microbiological cohorting
Segregate clinics into cohorts of *B. cepacia*, multi-resistant *Pseuodomonas aeruginosa* (PsA), other PsA, non-PsA, i.e. 4 clinic days.

Individual segregation
Segregation of all patients from each other during clinic visits; this accepts that knowledge of lower airway organisms is poor in many patients with CF who do not expectorate, and the safest approach is to assume that all patients may have organisms potentially cross infectious to others.

In this clinic model, patients are allocated an individual time for attendance, are provided with a clinic room which they remain in for their whole appointment and through which health professionals rotate to consult the patient (as opposed to the traditional model of patients rotating through rooms to consult health professionals). Clinic room surfaces are cleaned between patients, and health professionals must adhere to scrupulous cleaning of hands and instruments.

Box 2.4 Clinic review

Chest
Recent symptoms
- Cough/breathlessness/wheeze/sputum production/haemoptysis
- Recent antibiotics and response (or lack of).

Auscultation
- Crepitations are typically a feature of advanced, and often irreversible, CF lung disease, and significant respiratory infection often occurs in the absence of chest signs in patients with CF
- Wheeze may occur in those with concurrent asthma, secretions in the airways or allergic bronchopulmonary aspergillosis (ABPA).

Pulmonary function
- Spirometry at clinic visits. Loss of function should be as slow as possible. 10% reduction between visits considered important to regain, usually with intravenous antibiotics unless rapidly gained by oral antibiotics. Deteriorating pulmonary function may be slowed by use of mucolytics (i.e. DNase) in addition to regular chest physiotherapy and antibiotics.

Physiotherapy
- Adherence and technique should be checked and alternate techniques suggested if required
- Microbiological culture of cough swab or sputum.

Abdomen & nutrition
Weight and height (often as BMI)
- Plotted and reviewed for rate of change in children, and weight gain/loss in adults.

Recent symptoms
- Abdominal pain/discomfort
- Stool frequency and colour.

Palpation
- Faecal masses are most frequently palpated in the right lower quadrant – patients with chronic masses can often point them out to you.

Nutritional supplements
- Oral (often poorly tolerated/adhered to)
- Overnight or daytime bolus feeds may be given by nasogastric tube or via gastrostomy.

Diabetes
- Typically subtle signs. Diabetes may only be present during a respiratory exacerbation
- Suspect where there are increased respiratory infections and/or weight loss/poorer gain than expected, particularly in those over 10 years of age.

Liver disease
- Often not associated with symptoms and detected by abnormal liver function tests at annual review. Usually first palpated as a large liver. May be associated with varices and haematemesis, or portal hypertension with large spleen and abdominal discomfort.

Box 2.4 continued

Polyps/sinusitis
- Recurrent headache or frontal pressure
- Nasal obstruction
- Loss of sense of smell and taste.

Bone & joint disease
- Joint pain/reduced mobility
- Recent bone fracture
- Poor bone mineralization may occur in patients with CF with poor mobility (compounded by Vitamin K malabsorption). DXA scans and supplementation of Vitamin K and Adcal may help.

Clinic Microbiology review
- Oral antibiotics
  - Most commonly given at high dose for prolonged courses (typically 14 days) appropriate to the most recent and/or most frequently identified organism on sputum/cough swab culture.
- Intravenous antibiotics
  - Reserved for infection responding poorly to oral antibiotics or in those with regular sputum production/bronchiectasis or where there is a rapid loss of respiratory function (see Chapter 5).
- Long term antibiotics
  - Consider if persistent growth of organisms on cough swab or sputum (see Chapter 4).

2.4.3 Inpatient

Most admissions to hospital are for intravenous antibiotic therapy to treat a chest infection (see Chapter 5). The same cross infection concerns during out-patient contact apply also to in-patient care.

- Patients should be segregated and have no, or minimal, contact, and should not share the same area for physiotherapy without the area being cleaned and ventilated thoroughly.
- Patients and carers should perform handwashing when moving between areas.

2.5 Annual review

The patient with CF requires careful review at least once each year as the condition is both multidisciplinary and multisystem. Disease progression is often subtle and slow. Careful attention to detail may identify and impede acceleration in speed of decline.

The annual review enables members of the multidisciplinary team to reflect on the rate of change for systems individually and

Table 2.2 CF annual review – typical investigations

Blood samples
- Full blood count
- Urea & electrolytes, calcium, magnesium and phosphate
- Random blood glucose & glucose tolerance test
- Liver function tests
- Total IgE, specific IgE to aspergillus & aspergillus precipitins
- Other immunoglobulins: IgG, IgA, IgM
- Vitamin A, D, E and K
- Pseudomonas antibodies.

Pulmonary function
- Spirometry +/– reversibility to bronchodilator
- Lung volumes
- Transfer factor
- SpO_2 on air.

Exercise tolerance
- Measure of exercise tolerance (i.e. 6 minute walk or 3 minute step test).

Respiratory review
- Change in symptom frequency over past year (cough, respiratory exacerbation, perception of breathlessness)
- Number, frequency and type of antibiotic courses
- Sputum frequency, volume and colour
- Evidence of haemoptysis.

Microbiology review
- Type of organism, frequency of occurrence, change in sensitivity patterns.
- Culture for detection of unusual pathogens (aspergillus and mycobacteria).

GI/nutrition review
- Height and weight centiles/z scores with BMI
- Review of dietary intake with food diary
- Review of dose and frequency of pancreatic enzyme supplements
- Liver ultrasound (annually if abnormal liver function tests or as clinically indicated)
- Bone densitometry every 3 years from early teens.

Psychology & social review
- Review of psychological adaptation to disease and changes in condition during past year
- Is patient/family enabled to access benefits they are entitled to receive?
- Are schools/work places provided with sufficient information to sustain their continued support during periods of health related absence?
- Appropriate information on sexual health and reproduction
- Life expectancy and outcomes.

collectively, and consider how their discipline can modify outcomes in the subsequent year. This usually requires a systematic review of each of the systems affected by CF (see Box 2.4). Annual review is also a good opportunity to ensure that up to date screening has taken place for development of important complications (e.g. diabetes, osteoporosis).

2.5.1 Annual review outcomes

The annual review discussion should bring together the perspective of all disciplines and may include consideration of (but not limited to):

- Have unusual organisms been looked for?
- Should there be discussions about change in strategy for next year (for example – regular IV antibiotic treatment/trial of NG tube feeding etc)?
- Is rate of deterioration of pulmonary function greater than expected and does this warrant further investigation (CT chest, bronchoscopy etc)?
- Has consideration been given to age related issues, such as discussion for males on infertility and for females on need for contraception?

2.6 Transition

Children with CF grow up with a close cohort of multidisciplinary professionals providing care on a regular basis, where these professionals are a constant and (hopefully) friendly aspect of life for the nascent young adults as they approach the age of transition to adult services.

Transition to adult services is most often a significant wrench for parents, who have invested many years of faith in one group of professionals who then relinquish (often reluctantly) not only the close relationship with professionals, but also some degree of parental responsibility for ongoing care. See also Chapter 9 for a discussion of the psychological challenges of transition.

Young adults transition to adult services in a period between the 15th and 18th birthdays, most typically when 16–17 years of age.

2.6.1 The transition process

Age 12 years (depending on individual maturity)

Young adults should be encouraged to become more actively involved in providing details of symptoms and treatments.

Age 14 years onwards

Some young adults may benefit from seeing professionals on their own, with their parents joining consultations for a summary at the

> **Box 2.5 Transition process**
>
> **Visit 1** An initial transition clinic takes place with the paediatric team alone, where the process of transition is discussed, and young adults are invited to express their expectations and concerns.
>
> **Visit 2** Immediately preceding the second transition clinic, the two multidisciplinary teams meet to discuss the individual patients who are to transfer care that year, using a full written summary provided by the paediatrician. Pairs of professionals from each subdiscipline then go to meet the young adults with CF (and their parents) to review previous progress and to discuss a plan for future care (it is particularly important that transition is not associated with a step change in policy).
>
> **Visit 3** In the third clinic meeting a similar process occurs, but this time hosted by the adult care team at the adult unit, with the adult teams taking the lead during consultations.
>
> **Visit 4** In the fourth and final clinic young adults meet with the adult team at the adult unit, without a paediatric presence and the transition is considered complete.

end. Young adults can begin to be invited to participate more actively in healthcare decisions, and balancing the risk and benefits of choices.

Age 15 to 18 years

A formal process of transition takes place to transfer care to adult services. There are many models. In the UK, it is recommended that a process of transfer takes place over the course of four clinic appointments in a period of covering six months (Box 2.3).

At the completion of visit 4, no further advice or in patient care is directed by the paediatric team and the process of transition is considered complete.

References

Gibson L.E., Cooke R.E. (1959) A test for concentration of electrolytes in sweat in CF of the pancreas utilizing pilocarpine iontophoresis. *Pediatrics* **23**: 545–9.

Farrell P.M., Rosenstein B.J., White T.B., *et al.* (2008) Guidelines for diagnosis of cystic fibrosis in newborns through older adults: CF Foundation consensus report. *J. Pediatrics* **153**: S4–S14.

Castellani C., Southern K.W., Brownlee K., *et al.* (2009) European best practice guidelines for cystic fibrosis neonatal screening. *J.C.F.* **8**: 153–7.

Transition Medicine Clinical Standards. (2008) CF. Royal College of Physicians of Edinburgh (www.rcpe.ac.uk).

Chapter 3

Microbiology of CF lung disease

Gerd Döring and Dieter Worlitzsch

Key points

- Bacterial lung infections are the predominant cause of restricted life expectancy of CF patients
- Eradication of bacteria chronically infecting the CF lungs is virtually impossible
- Bacteria adapt their genotype and phenotype to the specific lung environment
- CF lung infection involves a mixed growth of facultative and obligate anaerobes
- Anaerobic growth conditions induce *Pseudomonas* biofilm formation, reduce the efficacy of the human defence system, and impair the effectiveness of antibiotics
- Early therapy at the onset of infection offers the best chance of eradication
- Many organisms are either innately resistant to multiple antibiotics or are able to acquire resistance.

3.1 Introduction

Respiratory infections start early in the life in CF and are the major cause of morbidity and mortality. Chronic pulmonary infections are caused by a surprisingly limited range of micro-organisms. Bacteria that usually cause severe pulmonary inflammation in healthy lungs, such as *Staphylococcus aureus*, may be relatively well tolerated. On the other hand, significant infections occur with organisms that rarely affect normal lungs.

Unlike the healthy lung, infections tend to be persistent, sometimes involving phenotypic change in the organisms themselves. Organisms may either colonize the lungs, not directly causing disease, or be responsible for uncontrolled infection and inflammation. Treatments are aimed at preventing acquisition or early eradication of new organisms. Eradication of chronic infection of many important pathogens, in particular *Pseudomonas*, is difficult if not impossible.

The sequence of infecting pulmonary organisms follows a classical chronological course, illustrated in Figure 3.1. In early childhood, *S. aureus* is the organism most frequently isolated from sputum/cough swab, with a prevalence of 50% by the age of 10 yrs. *Haemophilus influenzae* is also isolated frequently during childhood, but less so in older children and adults, in whom the major pathogen is *Pseudomonas aeruginosa. Stenotrophomonas maltophilia, Burkholderia cepacia* complex bacteria (BCC), *Achromobacter xylosoxidans,* and non-tuberculous mycobacteria (NTM) are commonly isolated. In addition, many species of obligate anaerobic bacteria have recently been identified in the airways of CF patients (Table 3.1).

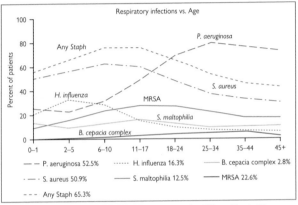

Figure 3.1 Age-dependent prevalence of bacteria in the CF lung. Used with permission from the Cystic Fibrosis Foundation Patient Registry. *2008 Annual Data Report.* © 2009 Cystic Fibrosis Foundation, Bethesda, Maryland.

Table 3.1 Major bacterial species in the CF airways	
Facultative anaerobic bacteria	Staphylococcus aureus
	Haemophilus influenzae
	Pseudomonas aeruginosa
	Burkholderia cepacia complex bacteria
	Stenotrophomonas maltophilia
	Achromobacter xylosoxidans
	Non-tuberculous mycobacteria, e.g. M. avium complex, M. abscessus, M. kansasii, M. simiae
Obligate anaerobic bacteria	Prevotella, Peptosteptococcus, Actinomyces, Staphylococcus, Veilonella, Clostridium, Bacteroides, Gemella, Capnocytophaga, Eubacterium, Lactobacillus, Mobiluncus, Propionibacterium, and Wolinella spp.

Microbiological methods

Laboratory techniques for CF microbiology are similar to those used for other chronic lung infections. Specific techniques, however, may need to be applied to address particular clinical questions, i.e. if the detection of the phenotypically different small colony variants of *S. aureus* or *P. aeruginosa* is requested, the agar plates have to be incubated for two days. Special culture media are required for the detection of mycobacteria and BCC organisms. In future, specific anaerobic culture techniques may be also be required.

3.2 Early infections

3.2.1 Staphylococcus aureus

Epidemiology

S. aureus is found in 51% of respiratory tract secretions of American CF patients, either as sole pathogen or in combination with other bacteria (Figure 3.1). Chronic *S. aureus* infection is particularly common in children. Family members of CF patients may share genetically identical *S. aureus* clones with patients, suggesting they may represent a source of *S. aureus* acquisition: 32% of healthy adults are nasal carriers of *S. aureus*, and rates of carriage are twice as high in CF. With increasing age, *S. aureus* is eclipsed by *P. aeruginosa* as the most commonly isolated micro-organism in the CF lung. However, small colony variants may be overgrown by mucoid *P. aeruginosa*; therefore the additional use of selective media for staphylococci such as mannitol salt agar or Columbia/colistin-nalidixic acid media is recommended.

Virulence factors

S. aureus isolates from CF patients may express several virulence factors: membrane-damaging toxins such as leukotoxins, hemolysins, or the Panton-Valentine leukocidin (PVL). PVL is a cytolytic toxin that forms pores in the membranes of leukocytes, leading to cell death. PVL is increasingly found in MRSA (meticillin resistant *Staphylococcus aureus*) strains. Surface factors and extracellular proteins (protein A, capsules) may inhibit phagocytosis, and enzymes such as superoxide dismutase may inactivate neutrophil-derived oxygen radicals and thereby impair innate antimicrobial defences. Small colony variants, so called because of their appearance on agar plates, are associated with greater persistence in the airways and greater adherence to respiratory epithelium.

Clinical consequence

S. aureus colonizes the lung early in life, and causes recurrent infection in some. Troublesome infection may require use of nebulized antibiotics.

Treatment

There are two possible approaches to *S. aureus* infection. The first is to provide prophylactic treatment to newborns with CF to protect against aggressive *S. aureus* infection, at least for the first 3 years, to reduce the prevalence of *S. aureus* infection and associated inflammation. Evidence for this approach is limited, and there are concerns that continuous antibiotics may predispose to a higher rate of Pseudomonas acquisition. The second approach is to regularly monitor airway secretions microbiologically and provide prompt treatment of symptomatic *S. aureus*. Treatment of acute exacerbations involving *S. aureus* is described in Chapter 5.

3.2.2 **MRSA**

MRSA bacteria exhibit extremely high levels of antimicrobial resistance; usually they are susceptible to vancomycin exclusively. Rates of MRSA detection have increased amongst American and UK CF populations, in line with increases in MRSA colonisation in the community. The *mecA* gene confers resistance to meticillin and is found with increasing frequency in CF patients' airways.

Clinical consequence

MRSA is associated with more frequent intravenous antibiotic courses, increased hospitalization and lower lung function values in CF children and adults. PVL is expressed more frequently by MRSA strains compared to meticillin sensitive *S. aureus*. PVL-positive patients are more likely to be hospitalized for pulmonary exacerbations, have more infiltrates on chest radiographs and a greater decline in lung function compared to CF patients with PVL-negative MRSA strains.

Treatment

Many centres now adopt an aggressive policy towards MRSA in CF, with multiple attempts at eradication. This is because chronic MRSA carriage may be problematic if the patient subsequently requires lung transplantation. A variety of eradication regimens are used in practice, and these can produce sustained eradication in over 50% of patients. Up to three attempts at eradication, using the same or different therapies, are recommended. An example of an eradication regimen is given in Box 3.1.

Nebulized vancomycin has also been used in eradication regimens in clinical trials. This is given 2–4 times daily for the first five days of treatment as 250mg (or 4mg/kg in children) diluted to 4ml in sterile water. Oral linezolid should only be used under supervision of a microbiologist, and its use is limited to 14 consecutive days. If anti-staphylococcal prophylaxis is also prescribed, this should be discontinued whilst the patient is on a MRSA eradication regimen, but can be restarted if eradication is successful.

Box 3.1 MRSA eradication regimen for CF patients	
1st line 6 weeks	• Rifampicin 5–10mg/kg (max 450mg) (children and adults<50kg), 600mg (adults) PO 12hrly • Fusidic acid 15mg/kg (<1yr), 250mg (1–5yrs), 500mg (5–12yrs) or 750mg (>12yrs) PO 8hrly.
2nd line 6 weeks	2 of the following antibiotics depending on sensitivities: • Doxycycline (>12yrs) 200mg first dose, then 100–200mg PO once daily • Trimethoprim 4mg/kg (max 200mg) PO 12hrly • Rifampicin* (see above for dosing) • Fusidic acid* (see above for dosing).
3rd line 2 weeks, followed by 4 weeks of a 2nd line combination	• Teicoplanin 10mg/kg (max 400mg) IV 12hrly for 3 doses then once daily OR • Linezolid 10mg/kg (max 600mg) PO 8hrly (<12yrs) or 600mg PO 12hrly (>12yrs)

*Rifampicin and fusidic acid should not be used together for this course; either can be combined with another antibiotic

Eradication also involves elimination of non-respiratory carriage. The following steps are recommended:

• Change bed linen, towels and toothbrush at start of eradication
• Replace all nebulization components
• Topical mupirocin 2% or vancomycin cream 2% to anterior nares twice daily for 5days
• 4% chlorhexidine bath/shower on alternate days
• Oropharyngeal carriage: vancomycin 5% lozenges qds or vancomycin 2% paste/gel qds.
• High level of hygiene and handwashing
• Immediate household contacts should be screened and those who are also colonized by MRSA should be treated in the same way.

3.2.3 Haemophilus influenzae

H. influenzae may play a major role in pulmonary infection in young CF children. Infection tends to be more acute/periodic and less chronic than that for other organisms. Detection of *H. influenzae* requires specific media such as chocolate agar (supplemented with bacitracin) incubated anaerobically. *H. influenzae* may chronically colonize the CF lung; penetration of the bacteria into epithelial cells may contribute to persistence of *H. influenzae* in CF. *H. influenzae* infection in CF patients is associated with increased inflammatory markers (CRP) during acute exacerbations and with high bacterial counts in sputum. Treatment of exacerbations due to Haemophilus must take account the presence or absence of beta lactamase producing strains, which will affect susceptibility to amoxicillin.

H. influenzae is associated with fewer pulmonary exacerbations in older CF patients. Strains that are found in the CF lung are unencapsulated. Application of the *H. influenzae* type B vaccine therefore does not protect from the acquisition of the unencapsulated CF strains.

3.3 **Pseudomonas aeruginosa**

3.3.1 **Background**

P. aeruginosa is a ubiquitous Gram-negative rod-shaped bacterium with one or more polar flagellae. It is found in many environments, including soil and water, and is an important opportunistic pathogen, primarily in those with impaired immunity. It is implicated in respiratory and urinary infections in particular, and is found in 10–20% of all hospital acquired infections.

P. aeruginosa possesses a large genetic diversity and a number of features that contribute to its ability to persist in the environment, and to its pathogenicity. It is intrinsically resistant to a number of antibiotics, is able to metabolize various carbon and nitrogen sources, and can grow in both aerobic and anaerobic environments. It also possesses a number of virulence factors, including LPS, pili, flagella, and secreted factors such as elastase and exotoxins.

Non-mucoid and mucoid forms

In the environment, *P. aeruginosa* exists as single motile bacteria that form rough colonies on agar plates. This is the so-called non-mucoid form of the organism. The pili bind to airway epithelial cells, permitting colonisation of the airways. *P. aeruginosa* stimulates the innate immune system, resulting in the production of cytokines responsible for neutrophil chemotaxis. Virulence factors are switched on by the organism's quorum sensing (QS) mechanisms. These are diffusible signalling molecules that allow the bacteria to respond to increases in cell density. Production of alginate, an exopolysaccharide which leads to aggregation of many *P. aeruginosa* cells into a matrix (biofilm), has been linked to decreasing environmental oxygen tensions and QS activation. This is the mucoid form of *P. aeruginosa*, so called because of the appearance of the colonies on agar plates.

Chronic infection of the CF lung

Children with CF infected with *P. aeruginosa* have poorer pulmonary function, lower chest radiograph scores, and lower 10 year survival rates than uninfected CF children, emphasizing the important role of this pathogen in CF. Pseudomonas forms biofilms which are more resistant than single bacterial cells to destruction by the innate immune system and therefore persist. Such chronic infection causes antibody production against numerous bacterial antigens, formation of immune complexes and creates large numbers of activated neutrophils in the airway lumen. Neutrophils unable to eradicate the persisting biofilm bacteria expire, releasing their contents of proteases and other toxins contributing to the cycle of airway destruction and remodeling. In addition, *P. aeruginosa* virulence factors, particularly secondary metabolites (e.g., rhamnolipid) or secreted protein toxins (e.g., elastase, alkaline protease, exotoxin A, exotoxin U, exotoxin S) are thought to further contribute to lung tissue damage.

3.3.2 **Routes of transmission**

Since *P. aeruginosa* plays such a dominant role in morbidity of CF patients, every effort should be undertaken to prevent acquisition, i.e. reducing routes of transmission from the environment to the patients. Direct patient-to-patient transmission occurs. Genotyping methods also suggest that transmission of Pseudomonas to CF patients occurs via contaminated environmental water reservoirs inside and outside of hospitals (Table 3.2). In particular, washbasin sinks can be contaminated. Handwashing at contaminated sinks without subsequent disinfection may lead to Pseudomonas-contaminated hands, allowing transmission either directly to patients or via hospital

Table 3.2 Routes of *P. aeruginosa* transmission		
Bacterial source	**General measures**	**Specific examples**
Patient-to-patient contact	Avoid close individual contacts, especially in hospitals	Divided clinical areas or treatment times for patients with different colonizing bacteria
Washbasin contamination (in hospitals)	Continuous supervision of the hospital water system, chemical or thermal disinfection	Installation of bacterial-dense filters in CF wards
Washbasin contamination (at home)	Individual hygiene	Cleaning of sink areas
Medical equipment	Single-use material, disinfection, sterilization, employment of dry equipment	Single-use tubing for lung function measurement, adequate sterilization of bronchoscopy equipment
Dental equipment	Disinfection of the water supply for dental units	Treatment of CF patients directly following disinfection, use of dental dam

personnel. Survival of mucoid *P. aeruginosa* is significantly prolonged compared to non-mucoid forms. Definitive proof that CF patients have been infected by a given contaminated environmental source are rare. Hygienic measures to decontaminate environmental reservoirs of *P. aeruginosa*, and hand disinfection for CF patients and hospital personnel, are considered vital to reduce transmission.

Patient segregation

To avoid cross-infection amongst patients, CF centres commonly separate CF patients with and without Pseudomonas infection. In many centres Pseudomonas-infected CF patients are seen on separate days of the week. Similar strategies are also recommended for the separation of other patient groups, such as for CF patients with antibiotic multi-resistant *P. aeruginosa* strains, B. cepacia complex strains or MRSA strains. In the Copenhagen CF centre, application of these methods has led to a decreased incidence and prevalence of *P. aeruginosa* infection. Summer camps and other social activities where CF patients live together for certain periods of time are generally discouraged.

3.3.3 Diagnosis

P. aeruginosa infections are typically diagnosed by obtaining sputum or throat swabs using routine microbiological culture. Serological tests for *P. aeruginosa* antigens (generally ELISA assays) may be useful in non-expectorating patients, including patients younger than 6 years, in whom routine Pseudomonas surveillance may yield false-negative results. The adaptive immune system of CF patients is not compromised, and an increasing number of bacterial antigens are therefore recognized by specific circulating antibodies during the course of the disease. These can be detected by ELISAs on patient serum. In some patients, the indirect detection of *P. aeruginosa* by ELISA precedes the detection of the pathogen by microbiological culture methods. In addition polymerase chain reaction (PCR)-based methods of bacterial DNA amplification have been used to detect bacterial pathogens in specimens from CF airways. There is increasing evidence that early diagnosis of Pseudomonas lung colonization is beneficial, since early antibiotic treatment can be initiated (see below). Therefore it is recommended that all CF patients, regardless of clinical status, should have a respiratory tract culture performed at least quarterly. The more frequently microbiological investigations are performed, the higher is the probability that first colonization with Pseudomonas is detected early, before the infection becomes established. In culture negative, symptomatic, non-expectorating young children bronchoscopic evaluation of the lower airway may be necessary to demonstrate infection with *P. aeruginosa*.

3.3.4 **Pseudomonas vaccines**

Prevention of *P. aeruginosa* infection might in future also be achieved by vaccination. However, a phase III trial using an exotoxin A-polysaccharide conjugate vaccine has been stopped because no significant benefit (compared with control) was seen in vaccinated patients. The efficacy of the Pseudomonas-flagella vaccine is not comparable to diphtheria or tetanus vaccines. There is no Pseudomonas vaccine on the market at present.

3.3.5 **Early eradication therapy for Pseudomonas**

Antibiotic therapy, initiated shortly after the confirmation of *P. aeruginosa* lung colonization, provides a very promising method of eradicating Pseudomonas infection before it becomes established. The bacterium exhibits the non-mucoid phenotype at the time of colonization, and eradication of the pathogen if treated at this early stage seems to be possible. Indeed, the combined treatment of aerosolized colistin and oral ciprofloxacin significantly reduced the onset of chronic Pseudomonas infection in treated CF patients compared to untreated controls. Similarly, a placebo controlled double-blinded, randomized tobramycin inhalation study showed that after onset of Pseudomonas colonization, the time of conversion to a *P. aeruginosa* positive respiratory culture was significantly prolonged by active treatment, suggesting that early treatment may prevent Pseudomonas pulmonary infection in CF.

Antibiotics used for eradication therapy are described in Chapter 4.

3.3.6 **Antibiotic therapy strategies**

It is virtually impossible to eradicate mucoid *P. aeruginosa* in the chronic infection state using any antibiotic therapy regimen, and at best this achieves only a reduction of Pseudomonas cell numbers. This phenomenon is explained by the highly reduced efficacy of nearly all antibiotics under reduced oxygen tensions. Hypoxic conditions in CF sputum have been confirmed in vivo by direct measurements of oxygen partial pressures in airways of CF patients. Oxygen diffusion through Pseudomonas biofilms is poor, creating hypoxic zones around the bacterial colonies. Sub-inhibitory concentrations of antibiotics in CF airways may negatively affect clinical outcomes by inducing Pseudomonas biofilm formation and increasing the rate of mutation of hypermutable strains.

However, reduction in bacterial cell numbers is still beneficial since it improves clinical outcome, reduces inflammatory parameters, increases quality of life, and improves nutritional status of the patients. Besides antibiotics, improved mucolytic therapy, more intensive airway physiotherapy and enhanced nutritional strategies have contributed to the increased life expectancy in CF patients. Due to the endobronchial location of mucoid Pseudomonas in anaerobic plugs, high doses of antibiotics are recommended to achieve satisfactory drug concentrations at the site of infection. To obtain sufficiently high antibiotic dosages in the CF lung, antibiotics such as tobramycin and colistin have been given by the aerosolized route, a strategy which reduces adverse effects compared with intravenously administered antibiotics. During acute exacerbation, antibiotics should also be administered intravenously (see Chapter 5).

3.4 Other important pathogens

3.4.1 Burkholderia cepacia complex (BCC)

Epidemiology

BCC is a group of Gram-negative bacteria comprising at least 9 distinct species, known as "genomovars" (see Table 3.3). These are phenotypically identical, require specific culture media, and are iden-tified on the basis of biochemical or DNA-based tests.

BCC are ubiquitous environmental organisms, commonly found in soil and water. They are particularly important in CF because of their innate antimicrobial multi-resistance, transmissibility and potential to induce a florid and life threatening inflammatory response.

Clinical consequence

In the last 15 years, BCC organisms have emerged as important pathogens in CF. *B. cenocepacia* and *B. multivorans* account for approximately 90% of isolates from CF sputum, and both may be associated with epidemic spread. The organisms are highly transmis-sible and new acquisition may lead to a rapid and irreversible decline in lung function. Clinical course commonly follows one of three patterns after acquisition:

1. No deterioration in lung function or clinical condition.
2. Accelerated decline in lung function (most common).
3. Rapid and fatal decline in lung function.

This last pattern may be accompanied by septicaemia and is known as the 'cepacia syndrome'. This is most commonly associated with *B. cenocepacia*, but is not exclusive to this genomovar, and may occur many years after acquisition. Patients chronically infected with stable BCC do not appear to have more frequent exacerbations than those infected with *P. aeruginosa* alone.

Infection with *B. cenocepacia* is considered a contra-indication to lung transplantation because of the higher rates of early post trans-plant mortality.

Genomavar	Species
I	B. cepacia
II	B. multivorans*
III	B. cenocepacia*
IV	B. stabilis
V	B. vietnamiensis
VI	B. dolosa
VII	B. ambifaria
VIII	B. anthina
IX	B. pyrrocinia
*Most clinically significant genomavars	

Table 3.3 BCC genomavars

Treatment

Antibiotic treatment of *B. cepacia* complex infections is difficult since the pathogen is generally resistant to many classes of antibiotics including aminoglycosides, quinolones, β-lactams and antimicrobial peptides. Some BCC produce a highly inducible β-lactamase and are capable of using penicillin as a sole carbon source. Combinations of antibiotics, according to the minimal inhibition concentrations, are recommended. Combinations containing meropenem are most likely to be successful, usually together with one or more of chloramphenicol, co-trimoxazole, tetracyclines, or piperacillin-tazobactam.

In some patients there appears to be spontaneous clearance of the organism, but this should not be assumed until at least three sequential good quality sputum cultures, over 12 months, have been clear of the organism.

3.4.2 Mycobacterial infection

Epidemiology

Non-tuberculous mycobacteria (NTM) have been detected in an increasing number of respiratory specimens from CF patients. In a prospective, cross-sectional study of the prevalence of NTM at 21 U.S. CF centres, the overall prevalence of NTM in sputum was 13%, with *Mycobacterium avium* complex (72%) and *M. abscessus* (16%) being the most common NTM. In an Israeli study, prevalence of NTM approached 23% of the CF patients, with *M. simiae* (41%), *M. abscessus* (31%) and *M. avium* complex (14%) being detected most frequently. In end-stage CF patients, the prevalence rate for NTM was 20%.

Clinical consequence

Although no significant short-term effect on lung function has been demonstrated in patients with multiple positive NTM cultures, an abnormal high-resolution computed tomography (HRCT) was predictive of progression. Multi-resistant NTM, e.g. *M. abscessus*, is a significant additional risk factor which may be a relative contra-indication to lung transplantation.

Specific treatment, tailored to microbiological sensitivities, should be considered in those with *M. abscessus*, those repeatedly positive for for NTM on culture, and those with progression of changes on HRCT. The clinical significance of NTM in CF needs to be further studied as do the long-term effects of treatment.

3.4.3 **Stenotrophomonas maltophilia**

Epidemiology

S. maltophilia is another ubiquitous Gram-negative organism, found in aquatic environments, soil and vegetation. It may be found in plumb-ing, including shower heads, taps and sinks and is widespread in the home and in hospital. It may infect immunocompromised patients and prosthetic devices.

Prevalence in CF has been increasing over the last 20 years, and is between 10–30%. It is more likely to affect those with poorer clinical condition, but can also be found in patients with good lung function. Other risk factors include female sex, older age and co-colonization of BCC.

Clinical consequence

The clinical significance of the infection is controversial, and *S. malto-philia* produce few obvious virulence factors. A large retrospective US study found no independent association between survival of *S. maltophilia* patients compared to all others, when stratified for lung function. In individual patients however it may be clinically significant.

Treatment

The optimal treatment of *S. maltophilia* remains to be established, and no treatment is indicated if the organism is considered to be a colonizer. Despite an increasing number of resistant strains, co-trimoxazole remains the drug of choice. Minocycline shows good in vitro activity against *S. maltophilia*, but clinical experience is limited and it is contra-indicated in children under 12yrs. There is also good sensitivity (80%) to doxycycline. *S. maltophilia* is inherently resistant to carbapenems (imipenem, meropenem) and most strains are also resistant to aztreonam, tobramycin, piperacillin-tazobactam, and colistin.

3.4.4 **Achromobacter xylosoxidans**

As with Stenotrophomonas, the opportunistic human pathogen *A. xylosoxidans* (previously *Alcaligenes*) has also been recovered from respiratory tract cultures of CF patients with increasing frequency over the last decade. Water reservoirs may serve as sources for CF lung infection. Transmissibility of *Achromobacter spp.* between CF patients has not yet been demonstrated. As a more specific detection media, MacConkey agar can be used. The pathogenicity of *A. xylosoxidans* for CF patients remains largely unclear, although an association with pulmonary exacerbations for *A. xylosoxidans* has been reported. The prevalence rate for *A. xylosoxidans* varies widely between centres, but may reach up to 8.7%.

Therapy of *A. xylosoxidans* poses major problems because of intrinsic multiresistance or fast development of new resistance. Combination therapy with two or three antibiotics according to the *in vitro* susceptibility testing is recommended.

3.4.5 Obligate anaerobes

Following the demonstration of microaerobic/anaerobic conditions in CF airways secretions, obligate anaerobes have been isolated in CF airways in a number of studies from different centres. Average colony counts of 5×10^7 bacteria/ml sputum demonstrate that the bacteria proliferate in the sputum, and are not simply the result of oral contamination.

The percentage of CF patients positive for obligate anaerobes is high: these bacteria are present in the sputum of 91% of all CF patients and are also detectable in BAL from children with CF. Prevalence of anaerobes in CF sputum is similar in children (82%) and adults (94%). Up to 51% of the strains tested are resistant to antibiotics that are frequently used in conventional CF therapy (e.g. ceftazidime), whereas the vast majority of the anaerobes are still susceptible to meropenem. Interestingly, a high percentage (49%) is also resistant to metronidazole, an antibiotic that is not usually employed in the therapy of CF lung infections.

The involvement of the obligate anaerobes in CF lung pathogenicity is still unclear. Therefore, it is too early to make a recommendation for a specific therapy against the obligate anaerobes. This may change if it can be demonstrated that a reduction of obligate anaerobic cell numbers follows treatment with antibiotics for which the specific anaerobes are susceptible, and also that this correlates with some measure of clinical improvement after exacerbations.

References

Döring G., Høiby N. (2004) Early intervention and prevention of lung disease in cystic fibrosis: a European consensus. *J. Cystic Fibrosis* **3**: 67–91.

Döring G., Meisner C., Stern M. (2007) A double-blind randomized placebo-controlled phase III study of a *Pseudomonas aeruginosa* flagella vaccine in cystic fibrosis patients. *PNAS* **104**: 11020–5.

Garber E., Desai M., Zhou J. et al. for the CF Infection Control Study Consortium (2008). Barriers to adherence to cystic fibrosis infection control guidelines. *Pediatric Pulmonology* **43**: 900–7.

Olivier K.N., Weber D.J., Wallace Jr. R.J., et al. (2003) Nontuberculous mycobacteria. I: Multicenter prevalence study in cystic fibrosis. *Am. J. Respir. Crit. Care Med* ..**167**: 828–34.

Park M.K., Myers R.A.M. Marzella L. (1992) Oxygen tensions and infections: Modulation of microbial growth, activity of antimicrobial agents, and immunologic responses. *Clin. Infect. Dis.* **14**: 720–40.

Ratjen F., Döring G. (2003). Cystic Fibrosis. *Lancet* **361**: 681–9.

Tunney M.M., Field T.R., Moriarty T.F., et al. (2008) Detection of anaerobic bacteria in high numbers in sputum from patients with cystic fibrosis. *Am. . Respir. Crit. Care Med.* **177**: 995–1001.

Worlitzsch D., Tarran R., Ulrich M., et al. (2002) Effects of reduced mucus oxygen concentration in airway Pseudomonas infections of cystic fibrosis patients. *J. Clin. Invest.* **109**: 317–25.

UK CF Trust infection control working group (2008). Meticillin resistant Staphylococcus aureus. CF Trust.

Chapter 4

Management of stable CF lung disease

J. Alastair Innes

Key points

- Aggressive treatment of specific lung infections improves prognosis
- Eradication of new *Pseudomonas* infection slows progression
- Nebulized DNase improves lung function in some patients
- Azithromycin and nebulized tobramycin can reduce the burden of infective exacerbations and improve lung function
- In advanced disease, oxygen and non-invasive ventilation may buy sufficient time for definitive treatment by lung transplantation.

4.1 Introduction

The progressive improvement in outlook for patients with CF in recent years reflects the adoption of a variety of pro-active treatment strategies, which together maintain good lung health throughout childhood and well into adult life. A fundamental early step was the recognition by Canadian clinicians of the clear link between good nutritional status and lung health in cystic fibrosis. Nutritional therapy sufficient to normalize body mass index clearly improves lung function (see Chapter 6).

This chapter outlines the respiratory treatments which have contributed to improved prognosis. Pulmonary interventions capable of slowing the progress of lung disease fall into two main categories; those improving the clearance of infected sputum, and those directed primarily at reducing the burden of inflammation and infection in the CF lung.

4.1.1 Clinical features

In early, mild disease, examination of the chest is normal. Cough is a prominent early symptom, and may lead to the false initial diagnosis of cough-variant asthma in a child. The cough is initially dry, but episodes of purulent sputum production soon supervene. Coarse crackles develop over the affected region and probably represent the presence of viscous secretions in small and medium sized airways. Wheeze is a feature in a minority of patients, some of whom may have coincident asthma (see below).

As time passes, features of chronic airflow obstruction develop, including a barrel-shaped chest, loss of cardiac dullness, reduced crico-sternal distance and paradoxical inward movement of the lower ribs on inspiration (indicating a low, flat diaphragm). Coarse crackles become generalized, and areas of scarring, most common in the upper lobes, may lead to patches of bronchial breathing with increased vocal resonance. By this stage, accompanying finger clubbing is almost universal.

4.1.2 Radiological features

The chest x-ray is normal in early life. The earliest changes are usually streaky infiltrates in the upper lobes, which may initially clear between infections, but later become persistent. As bronchiectasis develops, ring shadows and 'tram line' parallel lines radiating from the hila (indicating thickened bronchial walls seen from the side) may appear, but these classical appearances are relatively uncommon and the plain radiograph is notoriously insensitive to early bronchiectatic change. In established CF lung disease (Figure 4.1), there are increased coarse lung makings in all lung fields. Scarring in the upper lobes frequently results in elevation of the hilar shadows. A number of x-ray scoring systems, e.g. the Northern Score (Box 4.1), are used to quantitate CF x-ray changes to document progression over time.

Computed tomography is far more sensitive than plain radiographs for demonstrating early bronchiectasis. Thick walled airways are clearly seen, and CT also demonstrates mucus filled bronchi and bronchioles (Figure 4.2), air trapping and patchy infective infiltrates. CT is used increasingly to document and quantitate the extent of CF lung disease, but radiation dose precludes routine serial use. CT is particularly useful if invasive mycobacterial disease or aspergilloma is suspected. It may also yield clues to the anatomical source of a major haemoptysis as a prelude to bronchial angiography.

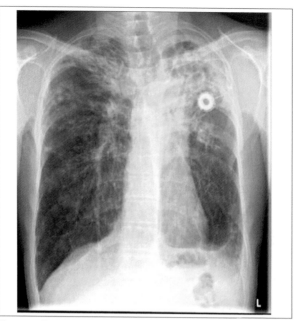

Figure 4.1 Chest X-ray in advanced CF. Note scarring and loss of volume in left upper lobe, also vascular access port on left chest wall.

Box 4.1 Northern Score: score each of the four quadrants 0–4 by the criteria below, and add a global score between 0 and 4	
Radiological changes	Score
Normal	0
Mild, minimal increase in linear markings and or nodular cystic lesions up to 0.5 cm in diameter	1
Moderate more pronounced linear markings and or more widespread nodular cystic lesions	2
Severe prominent increase in linear markings, profuse nodular cystic lesions, large areas of collapse consolidation	3
Very severe, little or no areas of normal lung seen, dense infiltration	4
Overall severity for CXR	0–4
Total score is out of a maximum (most severe) of 20	
Ref: Conway SP, Pond MN, Bowler I, et al. (1994) Thorax **49**: 860–2	

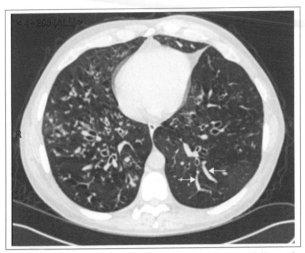

Figure 4.2 CT thorax in advanced CF. Note generalized thickening and dilation of the bronchi. Mucus-plugged airways are also seen in longitudinal section in the left lower lobe (arrows).

4.2 Physiotherapy

Effective airway clearance can be achieved in a variety of ways. A Cochrane review showed no clear difference in the efficacy of the various techniques, although patients expressed a preference for those which could be self-administered. Given the considerable investment of time and effort required of patients it is vital (in order to encourage adherence to treatment) that the technique which best suits that individual is selected.

4.2.1 Physiotherapy techniques

Commonly used techniques include:

- **Postural drainage and percussion ('conventional physiotherapy')**
  Gravity assisted positioning combined with chest percussion or vibration (manual techniques). This usually requires assistance from a second person and is most commonly used in infants and children. Caution is advised when using the head down position in those who have significant breathlessness or gastric oesophageal reflux. Manual techniques may not be appropriate in those with low mineral bone density.

- **Active cycle of breathing technique (ACBT)**
  A sequence of relaxed breathing followed by three to four deep breaths and forced expirations or 'huffs'. This may be performed independently in any position of comfort. Manual techniques may be incorporated into the breathing cycle.
- **Autogenic drainage (AD)**
  A breathing regimen using high expiratory flow rates at varying lung volumes. Performed independently in any position of comfort. AD may be combined with PEP or OPEP devices, as outlined below.
- **Positive expiratory pressure (PEP)**
  Exhalation into a mask or mouthpiece providing a positive pressure, thus splinting open the smaller airways to avoid early closure and potential trapping of sputum.
- **Oscillating positive expiratory pressure (OPEP)**
  Exhalation into a hand-held device, such as the Flutter® or Acapella®, which generates an oscillatory positive pressure. The vibratory effect is thought to reduce sputum viscosity. The Flutter only functions in the upright position whereas the Acapella may be used in any position of comfort.
- **External chest oscillation device**
  A mechanical device consisting of an inflatable jacket and air pulse generator that produces chest wall oscillation. Less common in UK compared to USA due to high costs and limited evidence base.

4.2.2 Exercise

Exercise may enhance sputum clearance and decrease breathlessness. Those with mild to moderate disease are generally able to exercise to the same level as their healthy peers. Those with more severe disease require careful assessment and supervised exercise programmes. Exercise is normally recommended in combination with postural stretches as part of a daily airway clearance programme.

4.2.3 Tailoring therapy to the individual

Once the appropriate airway clearance technique has been identified, it is important to coordinate the timing of inhaled medications around treatment sessions to ensure maximum benefit. Daily cleaning and drying of airway clearance devices and nebulizers is essential to avoid contamination of equipment.

Duration and frequency of airway clearance sessions will vary according to the patient's symptoms and lifestyle but some form of daily airway clearance technique is generally recommended in all patients. It is not uncommon for patients to be familiar with a range of techniques.

Positive pressure devices may be temporarily discontinued if certain complications arise such as significant haemoptysis or pneumothorax. Modification of airway clearance techniques may also be necessary during exacerbations and as the patient's condition deteriorates resulting in an increase in work of breathing. The application of non-invasive ventilation during physiotherapy may be necessary in those who are severely compromised in order to facilitate airway clearance.

Physiotherapy plays a key role in all stages of the disease, from teaching parents to perform techniques on their newborn baby through to palliation when a patient may choose to continue with some form of modified airway clearance to alleviate symptoms.

4.3 Drugs to aid secretion clearance

4.3.1 Recombinant DNase

The high viscosity of sputum in CF is believed to result in large part from the DNA released from dead neutrophils. Recombinant human DNase liquefies sputum in vitro by digesting the extracellular DNA molecules into smaller nucleotide chains. It is available as unit dose vials of 2.5mg for once daily nebulized administration. Several randomized controlled trials have demonstrated, in large numbers of patients, a mean improvement in FEV_1 of around 9% at 1 month, falling to 5% at 6 months. Some trials suggest a trend to reduced frequency of exacerbations in the treated patients however this is neither consistent nor statistically significant. Results are conflicting and the benefits less clear in patients with severe lung disease (FVC<40% predicted).

In practice, individual response is highly variable, with some patients gaining clear clinical benefit and others noticing no change. Because response in unpredictable, patients with productive cough are commonly given a 6 month trial period of DNase treatment after which they agree with their physician whether or not the benefits warrant continuation of treatment. Adherence to nebulized treatment may be improved if patients are offered modern vibrating-mesh nebulizers which can deliver the dose quickly and silently.

4.3.2 Hypertonic saline

Hypertonic saline can be administered by nebulizer with the aim of increasing the osmotic pressure of the airway lining fluid, drawing water into the airway. Early studies confirmed improved mucociliary clearance, though HS can cause cough and bronchospasm. A large controlled trial of HS (4ml of 7% NaCl nebulized twice a day over 48 weeks) showed only modest effects on FEV_1 (3.2% rise) but a marked reduction in the number of exacerbations and the number of days with exacerbation symptoms. Bronchodilator was used routinely prior to HS administration to prevent bronchospasm, but cough was still a significant adverse effect with HS treatment.

4.4 Airway infection and inflammation

4.4.1 Inhaled antibiotics

For CF patients with chronic airway colonization by *Pseudomonas aeruginosa*, nebulized antibiotics have been used for many years, particularly in Europe. The polymyxin antibiotic colistin is widely used in the UK by inhalation (usual dose 1–2 MU bd for an adult). Although studies have demonstrated a reduction in sputum bacterial load and improved symptom scores, large randomized trials showing functional improvement (e.g. improved lung function or reduced exacerbation rate) are lacking. A significant proportion of patients develop wheeze in response to inhaled colistin. The use of isotonic solutions and pre-treatment with beta-agonists can permit continued treatment in some patients.

Nebulized aminoglycosides have also been used in CF patients for many years, and a formulation of tobramycin specifically for nebulized use was tested against placebo in a large randomized US trial published in 1999. Tobramycin given 300mg bd by nebulizer alternate months increased lung function, and reduced hospitalization rates and the need for intravenous antibiotics compared to placebo. The medication was well tolerated and resistance to tobramycin did not appear to limit clinical efficacy.

Recommendations:

- In the UK, patients with chronic *P. aeruginosa* colonization are usually offered nebulized colistin 2 MU bd (1 MU bd for children) as first line treatment.
- Nebulized tobramycin 300mg bd alternate months is used for patients who are intolerant of colistin and those whose clinical condition deteriorates whilst receiving colistin.
- The first dose of nebulized antibiotic should be given in hospital with spirometry pre and post dosing in order to monitor for bronchoconstriction.

4.4.2 Oral macrolides

The striking efficacy of erythromycin in bronchiectasis associated with Japanese panbronchiolitis has prompted several large controlled trials of oral macrolides in CF in recent years. The precise mechanism of action of macrolides in bronchiectasis remains unclear. In stable laboratory cultures (as opposed to exponential growth cultures), macrolides appear to have bactericidal effects on *P. aeruginosa*. In addition, in vitro studies have demonstrated that macrolides can suppress pro-inflammatory cytokines and modulate neutrophil function.

A large randomized placebo-controlled trial of azithromycin (500mg oral 3 times a week; 250mg if <40Kg) in Pseudomonas-colonized CF patients was published in 2003. It demonstrated a modest mean improvement in lung function but a significantly reduced risk of pulmonary exacerbation compared to placebo, over the 6 month trial period. A further large placebo-controlled trial has extended these observations in a group of children, most of whom were not colonized with *P. aeruginosa*. In this year-long study a highly significant reduction in exacerbation rate was demonstrated.

This chronic oral treatment, normally given three times a week, is popular with patients as it is quick and convenient to take, and free of major side effects.

Recommendations:

- Regular oral macrolides (e.g. azithromycin 500mg 3 times a week (250mg if <40Kg)) should be considered in all patients colonized with PsA, particularly those deteriorating on conventional therapy, although they are sometimes withheld in patients with atypical mycobacterial infection to preserve their antimycobacterial activity.
- Evidence of benefit in those without Pseudomonas is much less strong, however a trial of treatment is reasonable in those with frequent chest exacerbations.

4.4.3 Inhaled steroids

The role of inhaled steroids in cystic fibrosis lung disease is contentious. The predominantly neutrophil-mediated inflammation in the airways of CF patients is believed to contribute to progressive damage to the airways over time, and oral corticosteroids do appear to reduce the progression of lung disease. The long term use of oral steroids is however precluded by adverse effects, particularly on skin, glucose tolerance, bone density and (in children) on growth.

Given the existing widespread use of inhaled steroids in CF, prospective trials of their effects are impractical to perform. A large multicentre randomized controlled trial of withdrawal of established inhaled steroid treatment has, however, shown that most patients receiving this treatment can stop it without any detectable decline in lung function or increased risk of exacerbation of their chest disease. Thus while there may be a small subgroup of patients with coincident asthma (see below) who do benefit from inhaled steroids, generalized prescription of these drugs to all CF patients is not supported by the evidence. The question of whether or not long term inhaled steroids might slow the decline in lung function with age has however not been investigated and would require a large and prolonged prospective trial.

4.4.4 **Other therapies**

Vaccination

Annual influenza vaccination should be offered routinely to all patients with established CF lung disease, as influenza may be associated with severe pulmonary exacerbations.

Exercise

Maintaining physical fitness in the face of CF lung disease is a challenge. There is evidence that exercise augments sputum clearance (see above). Deconditioning of the cardiovascular system and the peripheral muscles is common in advanced CF, due to inactivity and the effects of impaired nutrition. The residual exercise limitation seen after successful lung transplantation is one result. Deconditioning can be mitigated by a personalized exercise regimen during which patients with severe disease may require supplemental oxygen.

4.5 **Specific complications of CF lung disease**

4.5.1 **New sputum isolation of Pseudomonas aeruginosa**

The observation that cohorts of patients with airway colonization by *P. aeruginosa* are generally less well than their age-matched peers without Pseudomonas has led to the general assumption that early and aggressive eradication of first *P. aeruginosa* isolates may improve long term outcome in CF patients. Patients with Pseudomonas have a more rapid decline in lung function and chest x-ray scores, need more hospital days and courses of antibiotics and suffer impaired growth. Studies in this area are however plagued by the difficulty in distinguishing between the effects of the organism itself and its presence simply reflecting the presence of a more severe lung phenotype. Longitudinal evidence relating acquisition of *P. aeruginosa* to accelerated decline in respiratory health is conflicting; however standard clinical practice is now to make aggressive efforts with anti-pseudomonal antibiotics to eradicate *P. aeruginosa* following first isolation.

There are a number of small controlled clinical trials which confirm that it is possible using oral quinolones and/or inhaled tobramycin or colistin to eradicate *P. aeruginosa* from recently colonized patients for prolonged periods. The UK CF Trust recommends oral ciprofloxacin and nebulized colistin for up to 3 months (minimum of 3 weeks) as primary eradication treatment following first *P. aeruginosa* isolation (Box 4.2). Many centres also follow this with intravenous anti-pseudomonal antibiotics if cultures remain positive after oral and nebulized treatment. With these strategies, *P. aeruginosa* can be eradicated in the majority of cases, and it is now increasingly common for adolescent CF patients to undergo transition to adult services without chronic airway colonisation by Pseudomonas.

Box 4.2 Eradication of *P. aeruginosa*

- Nebulized colistin 1MU (<2yrs) or 2MU (>2yrs) 8–12hrly
  AND
- Oral ciprofloxacin: 15mg/kg (<5yrs); 20mg/kg (>5yrs); 750mg
  (adults), every 12 hrs for up to 3 months (minimum of 3 weeks)
- Inhaled tobramycin may be used in those showing early regrowth
  of Pseudomonas, or if intolerant of ciprofloxacin or colistin.

4.5.2 Asthma in CF

Asthma is a common condition, so it is not surprising that some CF patients also show features of asthma. The overlap between the symptoms of CF in the lung and those of asthma, and the fact that both conditions are characterized by bronchial reactivity, variable airway narrowing and infective exacerbations, complicates the precise diagnosis of asthma in CF. If bronchial reactivity is measured in CF using challenge testing, many patients exhibit periods of enhanced bronchial reactivity, particularly during and immediately after infective exacerbations.

Identifying patients with significant co-existing asthma is, however, important as they may benefit from specific asthma medications, in particular inhaled steroids. A history of atopy, hay fever or eczema together with wheeze as a prominent symptom are features suggesting an asthmatic component. Elevated total or allergen-specific (dust, pollen, animals) serum IgE levels and/or serum eosinophilia support the diagnosis, and if present a trial of oral or inhaled steroids is commonly given. Maintenance inhaled steroids are prescribed if symptomatic or objective benefit results.

4.5.3 Mycobacterial infection

Tuberculosis in CF patients may be missed because chronic upper lobe infection is a common feature of cystic fibrosis. A high level of suspicion is necessary to diagnose TB in this setting, and many units routinely check sputum samples once or twice a year to detect mycobacteria. Persistent fever or sweats despite adequate conventional antibiotic therapy, new or particularly cavitating lung shadows or progressive weight loss should prompt a thorough search for mycobacterial infection. CT scanning can be helpful in revealing cavitating disease. Standard treatment regimens for *M. tuberculosis* are effective in CF patients.

The airways of patients with CF are commonly colonized by non-tuberculous mycobacteria, particularly *M. avium*, *M. malmoense* and *M. abscessus*. In one study, sputum from 15% of patients attending US CF centres grew atypical mycobacteria. In the majority of cases, these non-transmissible strains of mycobacteria appear to be harmless colonizers of the airways and are not associated with new symptoms or radiological changes. Many patients clear the organisms spontaneously without specific treatment. A minority of patients, however, do develop persistent fever and new infiltrates with these organisms, and prolonged courses of multiple antibiotics, chosen according to sensitivity, are often needed to improve symptoms. *M. abscessus* is a particular problem when causing symptoms, as it is commonly resistant to multiple antibiotics. This organism has been associated with worse outcomes following lung transplantation and many centres may be reluctant to list patients colonized with *M. abscessus* for transplant. Treatment of atypical mycobacteria should be discussed with a microbiologist (see also Chapter 3).

4.5.4 Haemoptysis

The extensive bronchiectasis typical of CF lung disease is associated with hypertrophy of the bronchial circulation, predisposing to airway bleeding. Most CF patients experience minor haemoptysis at some stage in their life, usually in the presence of an infective exacerbation. Minor haemoptysis is nearly always self-limiting and patients should be reassured and treated in the conventional way for their airway infection. Treatment can also be offered with the pro-fibriogenic agent tranexamic acid (adult dose 0.5–1g up to 4 times daily)

A minority of patients develop intermittent episodes of brisk or major haemoptysis, which may amount to several hundred millilitres of blood, with an alarming feeling of choking or even suffocating. Episodes may occur with infection or spontaneously without warning. Patients should be nursed upright or with the affected side dependent if known. High flow oxygen is administered, intravenous access secured, clotting checked and blood cross-matched. Chest x-ray may reveal a new infiltrate indicating which lung is bleeding, and a CT scan may reveal abnormally enlarged bronchial arteries. Bronchoscopy in the acute phase is usually unhelpful due to the large volume of blood present throughout the bronchial tree. If bleeding persists despite correcting any clotting problem, patients should proceed urgently to bronchial arteriography (Figure 4.3) and therapeutic bronchial embolization.

In the hands of an experienced interventional radiologist, this procedure is often effective at stopping bleeding. It is common to find that large parts of the bronchial circulation in both lungs are abnormally dilated (Figure 4.3), and it is usually not possible to identify the bleeding point at angiography. Embolization of all affected dilated vessels may be attempted, though this can be difficult because of multiple vessel origins (intercostals, internal mammary and aorta). Great care must be taken to avoid obstruction of the anterior spinal artery, which often has a common origin with a bronchial artery.

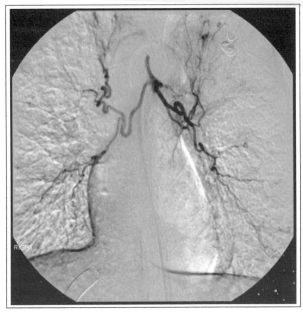

Figure 4.3 Bronchial arteriogram in a patient with CF and massive haemoptysis showing bilateral dilatation and tortuosity of the bronchial arteries.

4.5.5 **Pneumothorax**

The combination of extensive infective damage to the lung and the increased mechanical stresses due to airflow obstruction predispose CF patients to pneumothorax (Figure 4.4).

Although uncommon, pneumothorax in CF can cause serious additional impairment of respiratory function and may precipitate respiratory failure or occasionally empyema. Pneumothorax should always be considered in patients presenting with acute deterioration in their breathing. It may occur as part of an infective exacerbation; if not then the lung collapse itself will rapidly predispose to infective exacerbation. Either way the patient should receive appropriate antibiotics together with intercostal tube drainage for the pneumothorax.

Persistent air leak is a major problem for some CF patients with pneumothorax, as their underlying condition markedly increases the risks of surgical treatment. Every effort should be made to avoid surgery and achieve lung re-inflation by simple tube drainage, even if prolonged.

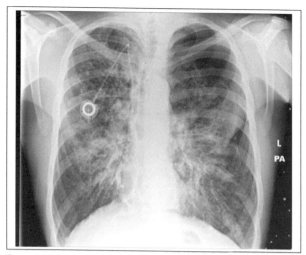

Figure 4.4 Left pneumothorax in a CF patient presenting with symptoms of acute exacerbation.

Clinicians are often concerned that pleurodesis procedures performed to treat pneumothorax may compromise patients' future chances of lung transplant surgery. In practice, surgeons generally advise that the priority should always be efficient and rapid resolution of the pneumothorax, including pleurodesis or apical pleural abrasion if necessary. Pleurectomy should, however, be avoided.

4.5.6 **Aspergillus in CF**

Airway colonisation by the ubiquitous environmental fungus *Aspergillus fumigatus* is very common in CF. The organism adopts a specific morphology only seen in CF, and in most cases appears to colonize the airways without causing harm. A small proportion of patients, however, develop allergy to Aspergillus with high blood levels of specific IgE, Aspergillus precipitins and eosinophilia. This may be associated with new x-ray infiltrates and worsening chest symptoms. As with allergic bronchopulmonary aspergillosis (ABPA) in asthma patients, treatment is directed at suppressing allergy using oral steroids, and suppressing the organism with antifungal agents. Itraconazole is commonly used in combination with prednisolone. Early reports suggest that the anti-IgE antibody omalizumab may have useful steroid-sparing benefits in CF patients with ABPA. Voriconazole is a highly active alternative antifungal agent which can also be used, however it can cause alarming side effects including anxiety, depression and hallucinations and this together with its high cost has inhibited its widespread use.

Diagnosis of ABPA

Diagnosis relies on a combination of the following criteria. IgE levels may be affected by systemic steroids and cutaneous reactivity by anti-histamines.

- Acute or subacute clinical deterioration, not due to another cause
- Serum IgE>500IU/ml
- Skin prick positive to Aspergillus antigens, or in vitro demonstration of Aspergillus-specific IgE.

AND at least one of:

- Aspergillus precipitins or specific IgG
- New or recent infiltrates or mucus plugging on CXR or CT, not responding to conventional therapy.

Recommendations:

- Standard initial treatment for symptomatic patients with proven ABPA and CF is prednisolone (0.5–1mg/kg/d, maximum 60mg) together with itraconazole. Prolonged therapy (months) is usually required to control symptoms. The dose is reduced after the first 1–2 weeks, and then tapered to the lowest possible, to minimize side effects
- Patients starting itraconazole should have liver function tests checked at the start of therapy, after 1 month, then 3 monthly.

4.5.7 Sinonasal disease

The electrophysiological defect of CF affects the entire respiratory epithelium, including the lining of the nose and nasal sinuses. Common manifestations of CF in the upper airway include nasal polyps and chronic sinusitis. Patients may present with symptoms of nasal obstruction, anosmia, persistent purulent discharge or facial pain from sinus infection and obstructed drainage. Polyps may be large, in which case surgical resection is usually indicated. For lesser degrees of nasal obstruction, nasal steroid sprays are often sufficient.

Infective sinusitis may cause severe pain and require intravenous antibiotic treatment. Surgical sinus drainage procedures occasionally help those with recurrent symptoms. Sinus problems persist following lung transplantation; indeed transplant immunosuppression may exacerbate the problem so patients newly free of lower respiratory problems may still be burdened with the need for intravenous antibiotics.

4.5.8 Chronic respiratory failure

In mild CF lung disease, hypoxia is the main gas exchange abnormality (type 1 respiratory failure). The problem first arises overnight when minute ventilation declines physiologically, and overnight monitoring of oxygen saturation is used to detect the problem. Oxygen concentrators fitted in the patient's home permit long term oxygen therapy, usually required overnight in the initial stages. Patients with exertional symptoms may be desaturating during exercise even if resting blood gases are satisfactory. Oximetry during treadmill walking can detect this problem and exercise tolerance should be compared with and without supplementary oxygen. Ambulatory oxygen can be provided using conventional portable cylinders or cylinders which can be filled at home from adapted oxygen concentrators. Oxygen conserving devices which release oxygen only during inspiration can significantly increase the duration of therapy available from small portable cylinders. Liquid oxygen is an alternative method of supply for home and portable oxygen therapy but is not universally available.

As disease progresses, type 2 respiratory failure with CO_2 retention eventually supervenes. Patients may notice morning headache, a symptom which should trigger measurement of morning blood gases. For patients with acutely elevated CO_2 and acidosis in the context of an acute infective exacerbation, non-invasive positive pressure ventilation (NIV) is effective and life-saving treatment. For those with chronic elevation of CO_2, home NIV is a useful option for supporting the patient pending a lung transplant, and can buy sufficient time for transplant to occur. Treatment is normally initiated in hospital, and in the early stages patients may find benefit using it only overnight at home.

The place of chronic non-invasive ventilation in the palliative treatment of end-stage CF lung disease in patients who are not listed for lung transplantation is more contentious. A careful clinical assessment of the individual patient's needs should be made and a frank discussion of the options with the patient and their family is always required. Some patients with high respiratory drive who are distressed by chronic breathlessness may find NIV helpful in the palliation of breathlessness, however other patients feel distressed and claustrophobic when presented with NIV apparatus, and prefer a pharmacological approach to the management of breathlessness.

4.5.9 Terminal care for advanced CF lung disease

Managing death with dignity in a young patient is extremely challenging for the whole multidisciplinary team. A key challenge in many cases is identifying the point at which the hope of a lung transplant rescuing the patient from respiratory failure is replaced by the need to change tack and palliate symptoms, recognizing that death is inevitable. Patients and families differ in the extent to which they welcome discussion of these issues, but team members must offer the opportunity for such discussions if they are wanted.

The clinical situation is usually that of a prolonged infective exacerbation which has failed to respond to appropriate antibiotics. The patient may be febrile, breathless and also frightened. They are often sleep deprived and also undernourished as appetite is inevitably poor at such times.

Ideally the decision to manage with predominantly palliative intent should be a positive one following an open discussion among the team, patient, and family. Each of the patient's treatments should then be re-evaluated using the question 'is this helping the patient's comfort?' Although antibiotics may not be containing the patient's disease, they may be controlling their sepsis and fever, and are often continued for symptomatic benefit. Oxygen is useful palliation for breathlessness in hypoxic patients, and intravenous fluids should be offered to prevent uncomfortable dehydration. Beyond this, any pain should be addressed with appropriate analgesia, then the focus should move to the optimal control of breathlessness, which is often the most frightening symptom.

Morphine is very effective palliation for breathlessness and the dose should be titrated upwards according to response. In very anxious or panicky patients, benzodiazepines may be added to alleviate distress. The goal of treatment is to avoid at all costs the situation where the dying patient is 'fighting for breath'. Careful empathetic nursing supervision and constant dose monitoring and adjustment are necessary to avoid this. Morphine syringe pumps are a useful option in some patients.

The best outcome is a peaceful sedated state where the patient is still able to communicate freely with their family between periods of rest and sleep.

References

Balfour-Lynn I.M., Lees B., Hall P., et al. (2006) Multicenter randomized controlled trial of withdrawal of inhaled corticosteroids in cystic fibrosis. Am. J. Respir. Crit.Care Med. 173(12): 1356–62.

Bott J., Blumenthal S., Buxton M., et al. (2009) Guidelines for the physiotherapy management of the adult, medical, spontaneously breathing patient. Thorax 64: i1–i52.

CF Trust Antibiotic Working Group (2009) Antibiotic treatment for cystic fibrosis. CF Trust. May 2009.

Elkins M.R., Robinson M., Rose B.R, et al. (2006). A controlled trial of long-term inhaled hypertonic saline in patients with cystic fibrosis. N. Engl. J. Med. 354: 229–40.

Jones A.P., Wallis C. (2003) Dornase alfa for cystic fibrosis. Cochrane Database of Systematic Reviews 2010, Issue 3. Art. No.: CD001127. DOI: 10.1002/14651858.CD001127.pub2

Ramsey B.W., Pepe M.S., Quan J.M., et al. (1999) Intermittent administration of inhaled tobramycin in patients with cystic fibrosis. Cystic Fibrosis Inhaled Tobramycin Study Group. N. Engl. J. Med. 340: 23–30.

Saiman L., Marshall B.C., Mayer-Hamblett N., et al. (2003) Azithromycin in patients with cystic fibrosis chronically infected with Pseudomonas aeruginosa: A randomized controlled trial. JAMA 290:1749–56.

Chapter 5

Management of respiratory exacerbations

Alex Horsley

Key points

- Early recognition and treatment of CF exacerbations is one of the cornerstones of modern CF care
- Diagnosis is essentially clinical, based largely on patient symptoms
- Anything other than very mild exacerbations requires intravenous antibiotics, typically for 10–21 days
- Choice of antibiotics should be based upon known antimicrobial sensitivities
- Monotherapy should be avoided in *Pseudomonas* infections
- In patients colonized with *Pseudomonas*, treatment usually involves a combination of a β-lactam antibiotic and an aminoglycoside
- Treatment can be delivered at home but requires the same assessment as for inpatients, and close monitoring
- Treatment is multidisciplinary and also involves attention to physiotherapy, nutrition and glucose homeostasis
- Antibiotic hypersensitivities are common, particularly in those with repeated courses of treatment. Antibiotic desensitization can be attempted for each course if necessary.

5.1 Presentation and assessment

CF lung disease is characterized by recurrent episodes of increased pulmonary symptoms, termed exacerbations. These episodes are important events in the natural history of CF, with a significant impact on lung function, quality of life and mortality. Early resort to intravenous (IV) antibiotic therapy to treat new respiratory symptoms is one of the most important features of modern management of CF.

5.1.1 **Pathophysiology**

Little is known about the underlying pathophysiology of these events, which appear to be largely a result of increased endobronchial bacterial burden, rather than to the acquisition of new bacterial strains. Alterations in host defences (e.g. secondary to preceding viral infections) may also play a role. There is a spectrum of severity, from mild exacerbations with little objective evidence of inflammation, to severe and life threatening pulmonary sepsis. In the majority of cases however, the inflammatory response is largely restricted to the lung, with an increase in sputum inflammatory mediators but relatively little systemic inflammation.

Prevention and early treatment of pulmonary exacerbations is one of the key aims of effective management of CF. In order to reduce morbidity and mortality, this requires early recognition of a change in symptoms and aggressive management, usually with intravenous antibiotics, airway clearance and nutritional support.

5.1.2 **Diagnosis**

Despite the central role of exacerbations in the clinical course CF, there is no universally agreed definition of what constitutes an exacerbation. In research studies, a number of different scoring systems have been devised that combine patient symptoms with clinical evaluation and data from laboratory and lung function assessments.

The symptoms and signs most predictive of an exacerbation are increased cough, change in sputum volume or consistency (i.e. darker or thicker), decreased appetite or weight, and change in respiratory examination or rate. Ultimately, in the absence of an agreed definition, the diagnosis remains essentially clinical, and typically relies on the presence of three or more of the signs or symptoms listed in Table 5.1. Of these, symptoms are the most important, and isolated changes in lung function, radiology, or laboratory findings should prompt further evaluation to identify the cause. In young children, who do not typically produce sputum and cannot perform spirometry, exacerbations are much harder to diagnose and may be indicated by new onset cough, a decrease in weight-for-age percentile, or development of new respiratory signs.

5.1.3 **Mild exacerbations**

There is a wide range of clinical severity, and some well patients with mild or minimal symptoms will only require outpatient treatment with oral antibiotics. The presence of constitutional upset, or

Table 5.1 Signs and symptoms associated with pulmonary exacerbation

Pulmonary signs and symptoms (new or increased)

Exertional dyspnoea or reduced exercise tolerance*

Cough*

Wheeze

Change in sputum production:

  Volume*

  Appearance

  Colour (usually darker)*

  Consistency (usually thicker)*

Haemoptysis

Increased respiratory rate*

Change in respiratory examination:*

  Retractions or use of accessory muscles

  Change in chest sounds

Decreased lung function:

  Fall in FEV_1 by $\geq 10\%$ over usual baseline

Upper respiratory tract symptoms

Sore throat/coryza

Sinus pain or tenderness

Change in sinus discharge

Constitutional signs and symptoms

Malaise/fatigue

Fever

Decreased appetite/anorexia*

Weight loss*

Work/school absenteeism

Investigations

New CXR changes

Reduced oxygen saturations

Increase peripheral blood neutrophil count ($\geq 15 \times 10^9 l^{-1}$)

Those indicated by a * are those most strongly associated with a diagnosis of exacerbation.

Adapted from Ferkol et al. (2006).

changes in clinical examination or radiology, necessitates intravenous therapy. Some patients will present with upper respiratory tract symptoms alone (e.g. coryza and cough), but these viral infections can perturb host defences and progress to more severe respiratory symptoms if untreated. These can usually be treated as mild exacerbations with an antibiotic that will cover both *Staphylococcus aureus* (SA) and *Haemophilus influenzae* (HI) (e.g. oral co-amoxiclav), after sending appropriate microbiological samples.

Box 5.1 Assessment of patient

In patients being evaluated for intravenous antibiotics, the following assessments are recommended:

- Full clinical exam, paying particular attention to:
  - Temperature
  - Respiratory rate
  - Oxygen saturations
  - Evidence of increased respiratory effort in young children
- Sputum microbiology, or cough swab if not producing sputum (see Chapter 3)
- Spirometry
- Blood tests, including full blood count, electrolytes, liver function, CRP and blood glucose.
- Chest X-ray if:
  - suspected PTX
  - suspected lung collapse/consolidation
  - disproportionate breathlessness or hypoxia
  - failure to respond to therapy
- Consider ABG/CBG in advanced disease to exclude CO_2 retention.

In young children and infants, it may not be possible to perform lung function assessments, and chest X-ray is not usually indicated in most exacerbations.

5.1.4 **Epidemiology of exacerbations**

Frequency of exacerbations increases with age and deteriorating lung function, from 23% patients/year for children under 6 years to 63% for those aged 18 years and over. Other factors associated with an increased frequency of exacerbations include infection with *Pseudomonas aeruginosa* (PsA), reactive airway disease, viral infections, lower socioeconomic status and air pollution.

5.2 **Treatment of an exacerbation**

5.2.1 **Principles of treatment**

There are few randomized clinical trials to guide choice of therapy but the following principles are generally applied:

- There should be a low threshold for starting IV antibiotics
- Treatment involves the use of more than one antibiotic, in order to reduce the development of bacterial resistance to monotherapy

- The selected antibiotics should have different modes of action, e.g. a β-lactam and an aminoglycoside, in order to improve response by antibacterial synergy
- Treatment typically lasts 10–21 days, and decision to finish the course is guided by clinical response. Shorter courses may be insufficient to treat the infection effectively but reduce the burden for the patient, increase compliance, and reduce risk of toxicity
- Antibiotic choice should be guided by antimicrobial sensitivity testing of a recent sputum sample. If none are available, choice should be based upon knowledge of the usual susceptibilities of the colonizing organisms, or previously effective treatments. In vivo response is often poorly predicted by in vitro testing, and demonstration of resistance in the lab does not necessarily mean that antibiotic will be ineffective when given to the patient, especially if they have responded to it previously. There is insufficient evidence to determine the effects of combined antimicrobial sensitivity testing on clinical outcome (i.e. testing the effects of more than one antibiotic on bacterial cultures) and this is not widely available.

5.2.2 Elective versus symptomatic treatment

Some units apply a policy of regular (elective) antibiotic treatment, usually every 3 months, irrespective of clinical condition. The rationale is that this reduces the bacteriological burden in the lung, and reduces exacerbations and need for unplanned therapy. There is a theoretical risk of increased resistance if antibiotics are given more frequently. Studies on this are limited, but there is no evidence of a difference in clinical outcomes between elective and symptomatic antibiotics. In the absence of evidence, the decision to employ the elective approach is down to patient preference, and may be useful in those with frequent exacerbations or complex social circumstances.

An alternative use of elective antibiotics is immediately before events that are important to the patient (e.g. holidays, exams). This helps to avoid untimely therapy and ensure that they remain well for the event.

5.2.3 Routes of delivery

Antibiotics can be given orally, intravenously and/or nebulized. Oral antibiotics alone are reserved for mild infections, and significant exacerbations are typically treated using intravenous antibiotics. Nebulized antibiotics are used as maintenance therapy in patients chronically infected with PsA, and as part of the eradication regimen for PsA when first isolated (see Chapter 4). Their role in the treatment of acute exacerbations is less clear, but they are not usually employed in this role. Regular nebulized antibiotics should be continued whilst on IV antibiotics, unless the nebulized drug is also prescribed for IV treatment (e.g. tobramycin) in which case the nebulized drug is usually discontinued until the IV treatment is completed in order to avoid excess drug accumulation and toxicity.

5.2.4 Home treatment

Home intravenous antibiotic treatment (HIVT) is a practical and effective alternative to inpatient administration. There is an added burden on the patient or parent, who must be taught to administer the antibiotics themselves (typically requiring two or three days of inpatient education and supervision). This is offset by the advantages and freedoms of being at home, and overall there is no difference in QoL, or clinical outcomes, between HIVT and inpatient antibiotics.

To reduce the burden to patients, some units now offer pre-prepared IV medications, delivered to the patient's home.

Recommendations:

- Patients undergoing HIVT must be assessed by a doctor or clinical nurse specialist, as for any patient being admitted for treatment, including height, weight and lung function
- Patients/carers must have previously undergone training in HIVT, and be competent to carry this out. If not previously taught, a 2–3 day admission for intensive education and supervision is required
- Administration is either via a totally inplantable venous access device (TIVAD) or a long line (see below)
- The first dose is given under supervision in the unit. If a patient has not previously being exposed to the antibiotic, the first dose, and often the second, must be given in the unit. The patient should remain for 30–60 minutes after administration to watch for development of an allergic reaction
- Patients/carers should be provided with an anaphylaxis kit, and given clear written instructions in case of adverse reaction
- Patients should be followed up at least every 7 days, ideally with a home visit from a specialist nurse
- Patients may need to attend for serum drug levels and will need to be instructed when to do this. Ensure that contact details are recorded so that advice on subsequent dosing or blood tests can be passed back to the patient
- If the patient fails to improve, or adherence is poor, they should return to the unit for admission
- At the end of treatment, patients will need to return to the unit for assessment (including weight and lung function) to ensure success of treatment and removal of any lines.

5.2.5 IV access devices

1. Long lines

Long lines are inserted into a large peripheral vein, usually in the antecubital fossa. The catheter is long enough to access the larger, more proximal veins. They are usually left in for the duration of treatment, and can remain in place for up to 4 weeks, unlike small peripheral cannulae which typically require re-insertion every few days. They should be considered in those starting IV antibiotics who do not possess a TIVAD (see below). They should be flushed with heparinized saline after use. PICC lines (peripherally inserted central catheters) are similar, though longer, in order to access central veins. PICC line insertion requires special training and radiological confirmation of position.

2. Totally implantable vascular access device (TIVAD)

TIVADs, or 'ports', facilitate long term IV access, avoiding repeated peripheral venous cannula insertion and the irritant effect of infusions on small peripheral veins. A TIVAD consists of a silicone membrane, mounted in a titanium chamber, and inserted subcutaneously, usually on the chest wall (see Figure 5.1). The chamber is connected to a catheter tunnelled into a central vein. The device is inserted as a day case procedure, usually under local anaesthetic, by a vascular surgeon or anaesthetist. Venous access is achieved via a Huber (or 'gripper') needle inserted into the chamber through the skin and underlying silicone membrane. The Huber needle remains in place throughout the course of treatment, allowing repeated administration of IV therapies, whilst permitting almost unlimited physical activity.

TIVADS are generally well received by patients, but complications can develop and the mean survival of an individual port is around 3–5yrs. Complications occur in around 40%, most commonly catheter occlusion (20% of all TIVADs). Other complications include infection (9%, requiring removal in 80% cases), vascular thrombosis (5%), and catheter displacement (3%) or dis-insertion (2%). Blood sampling via the TIVAD is convenient for patients, but increases risk of thrombosis (relative risk 2.2). Occlusion or thrombosis can be diagnosed by injecting contrast dye during X-ray screening (a "line-o-gram"). Incomplete thrombotic occlusion can sometimes be relieved by urokinase infusion.

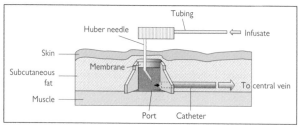

Figure 5.1 Huber needle inserted into TIVAD.

Recommendations:
- TIVAD should be considered in patients requiring IV antibiotics on a regular basis (i.e. more than 3 times per year), or those with difficult IV access
- Devices must be flushed every 4 weeks with heparin solution (5ml of 100iu/ml)
- Patients should be warned to seek advice if their TIVAD becomes slow to flush
- If possible, venepuncture should ideally be from a separate, peripheral, vein. In children, this is rarely possible
- Antibiotic levels must never be taken from a TIVAD.

5.3 Antibiotic selection

5.3.1 Pitfalls of antibiotic use in CF

Metabolism and clearance of some antibiotics is altered in CF, and the doses required to achieve therapeutic plasma levels are different from non-CF patients (see Chapter 3). Repeated dosing can lead to cumulative toxic effects (e.g. renal function and hearing impairment with aminoglycosides), and to the development of hypersensitivity. Gentamicin is no longer recommended in CF because of its association with renal failure, and tobramycin is the preferred aminoglycoside. This must be balanced against evidence showing that more aggressive and early use of antibiotics results in better preservation of lung function.

There is uncertainty as to the optimal antibiotic regimen at different stages of CF lung disease, and local guidelines may differ. The primary aims are to select the most effective and least toxic regimen, and the secondary aims are to choose the most cost-effective treatment and avoid the development of antibiotic resistance. Table 5.2 shows the typical antibiotic sensitivities of the common infecting organisms in CF. The choice of antibiotics will depend on the known, and likely, infecting organisms, and the clinical severity of the infection.

Children

For children who have never cultured PsA, or who have had repeated negative cultures for over 12 months following PsA eradication therapy, a suggested approach to antibiotic selection is given in Figure 5.2.

The presence of PsA should be suspected in children who have failed to respond well to two courses of non-PsA therapy, or in whom there has been a recent clinical deterioration. A concerted effort to obtain relevant airway cultures is necessary in these cases, either by induced sputum or bronchoalveolar lavage. A suggested approach to antibiotic selection in children with confirmed PsA colonization is illustrated in Figure 5.3.

Table 5.2 Antibiotic spectrum of activity					
Type	Antibiotic	Cover			
		SA	HI	PsA	BCC
β-lactam penicillin*	Flucloxacillin				
	Amoxicillin				
	Co-amoxiclav				
Cephalosporin	Cefuroxime				
	Cefotaxime				
	Ceftazidime				
Fluoroquinolone	Ciprofloxacin	+			
Anti-pseudomonal β-lactam	Piperacillin/ Tazobactam				
	Aztreonam				
	Meropenem				
Polymixins	Colistin				
Aminoglycoside	Tobramycin	+			
	Amikacin				

SA Staphylococcus aureus (not MRSA)

HI Haemophilus influenzae

PsA Pseudomonas aeruginosa

BCC Burkholderia cepacia complex

Dark shaded boxes indicate usually good antibiotic cover, and pale boxes indicate some activity against the organism. Unfilled boxes indicate no useful antibacterial activity. This is intended only as a general guide and should be checked against local and individual antibiotic sensitivities.

* These agents should not be used in severe exacerbations

+ Not suitable as monotherapy

Adults

PsA infection is common in older children and adults, and the use of monotherapy for intravenous medicines in these patients may encourage resistance and permit a selective bias, allowing the organisms to become established. Adult patients therefore are usually treated with antibiotics that also provide cover against PsA. A suggested approach is illustrated in Figure 5.4.

5.3.2 Identification of infecting organism

It is important to have up to date microbiological culture of respiratory tract samples in order to guide appropriate antibiotic selection and to monitor for the development of new infecting organisms. Few young children, and not all adult patients, can produce sputum

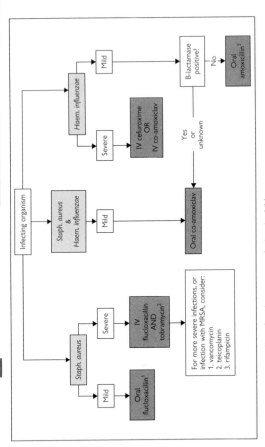

Figure 5.2 Treatment of non-*Pseudomonas* exacerbations in children

1: Alternatives include clarithromycin and erythromycin.

2: If tobramycin or other aminoglycosides can no longer be used due to bacterial resistance or intolerable side effects, IV colistin is a suitable alternative.

3: Cefaclor or cefixime if penicillin allergic. Cephradine and cefalexin not suitable. Doxycycline is another alternative if patient over 12yrs.

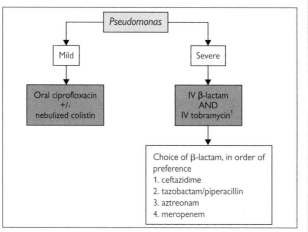

Figure 5.3 Treatment of exacerbation in children with *Pseudomonas*
1: If tobramycin or other aminoglycosides can no longer be used due to bacterial resistance or intolerable side effects, IV colistin is a suitable alternative.

spontaneously, even during an exacerbation. Alternative methods of sampling the respiratory tract include:

- Cough swab or plate
- Laryngeal or nasopharyngeal aspirate
- Bronchoalveolar lavage
- Induced sputum.

Recommendation:

Appropriate cultures should be obtained at every clinic visit and prior to starting antibiotics.

5.4 **Pharmacopeia**

The following section is intended as a quick reference guide. For full details on dosing and side effects, please refer to a local or national formulary.

5.4.1 **Exacerbations caused by *S.aureus* alone**

- **Flucloxacillin**
  - *Dose*: Child 50mg/kg 6hrly IV

    Adult 2–3g 6hrly IV
  - *Type*: β-lactam penicillin (inhibits synthesis of bacterial cell walls)
  - *Side effects*: GI upset, hypersensitivity
  - *Spectrum of action*: Main use is against SA.

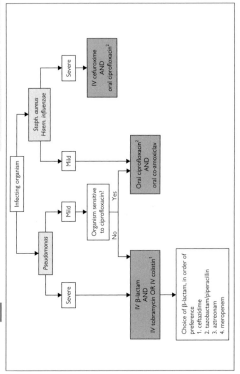

Figure 5.4 Treatment of exacerbation in adults

Other antibiotics may be prescribed on occasion, depending on microbial sensitivities and patient allergies.

If *Burkholderia cepacia* or *Stenotrophomonas maltophilia* are cultured from a patient's sputum, the above flowchart does not apply.

1: If tobramycin or other aminoglycosides can no longer be used due to bacterial resistance or intolerable side effects, IV colistin is a suitable alternative.

2: Oral ciprofloxacin is included in regimens where SA is the predominant organism in order to discourage the selection and enhancement of early cryptic PsA colonisation in these patients

Alternatives for treatment of meticillin sensitive SA:
- Clarithromycin
- Erythromycin.

Alternatives for treatment of MRSA:
- Doxycyline (not licensed under 12yrs)
- Vancomycin
- Teicoplanin
- Rifampicin (not as monotherapy)
- Linezolid – only after discussion with microbiologist.

5.4.2 Exacerbations caused by H. influenzae
- Amoxicillin/clavulanic acid (co-amoxiclav)
  - *Dose:* Child 25mg/kg amoxicillin IV tds or qds
    Adult 1.2g IV tds
  - *Type:* Penicllin (amoxicillin) combined with a beta-lactamase inhibitor (clavulanic acid)
  - *Side effects:* Hypersensitivity, GI upset, hepatitis, cholestatic jaundice
  - *Spectrum of action:* Active against SA and HI.
- **Cefuroxime**
  - *Dose:* Child 50mg/kg (max 1.5g) 6–8hrly IV
    Adult 750–1.5g 6hrly IV
  - *Type:* 2nd generation cephalosporin (inhibits bacterial cell wall synthesis)
  - *Side effects:* Diarrhoea, *Clostridium difficile* infection in adults, nausea, vomiting, headache, allergic reactions and blood dyscrasias.
- **Cefotaxime**
  - *Dose:* Child 50mg/kg 6–8hrly IV (max 12g/d)
    Adult 2g 8hrly IV (max 12g/d)
  - *Type:* 3rd generation cephalosporin
  - *Side effects:* see cefuroxime.
  - *Spectrum of action:* Should not be given as monotherapy – combine with aminoglycoside. Little activity against SA.

5.4.3 Exacerbations caused by P. aeruginosa
- **Ciprofloxacin**
  - *Dose:* Child <5yrs 15mg/kg 12hrly PO
    Child 5–18yrs 20mg/kg (max 750mg) 12hrly PO
    Adult 750mg 12hrly PO, or 400mg 12hrly IV
  - *Type:* Fluoroquinolone (inhibits DNA gyrase, necessary to separate replicated DNA, thereby inhibiting cell division)

- *Side effects*: Nausea, vomiting, joint pain, abdominal pain, headache, rash, dizziness, pruritis and hepatitis. A photosensitive rash is relatively common – avoid exposure to strong sunlight. Use with caution in epileptics
- *Spectrum of action*: Less effective against gram positive organisms, and high incidence of resistance in SA (should not be used as monotherapy against SA).

- **Piperacillin/tazobactam**
  - *Dose*: Child 90mg/kg (max 4.5g) every 6–8hrs IV
        Adult 4.5g every 6–8hrs IV
  - *Type*: Extended spectrum beta-lactam antibiotic (piperacillin) combined with a beta-lactamase inhibitor (tazobactam)
  - *Side effects*: Hypersensitivity, GI upset, transient hepatitis, cholestatic jaundice blood dyscrasias
  - *Spectrum of action*: Active against SA, HI and PsA.

- **Ceftazidime**
  - *Dose*: Child 50mg/kg 8hrly IV (max 6g/d)
        Adult 2–3g tds IV (max 9g/d)
  - *Type*: Third generation cephalosporin
  - *Side effects*: Rash, hypersensitivity, GI upset, diarrhoea, headache, dizziness, bad taste
  - *Spectrum of action*: See cefotaxime. No useful activity against SA.

- **Aztreonam**
  - *Dose*: Child 50mg/kg (max 2g) 6–8hrly IV
        Adult 2g 6hrly IV
  - *Type*: β-lactam antibiotic
  - *Side effects*: GI upset, rash, blood dyscrasias, hepatitis. Lower incidence of anaphylaxis than other β-lactams
  - *Spectrum of action*: Ineffective against gram positive organisms or anaerobes, but effective against PsA and HI.

- **Meropenem**
  - *Dose*: Child 25–40mg/kg (max 2g) 8hrly IV
        Adult 2g 8hrly IV
  - *Type*: β-lactamase resistant broad spectrum β-lactam
  - *Side effects*: GI upset, rashes, angioedema, blood dyscrasias, headache
  - *Spectrum of action*: Avoid use as monotherapy. Risk of increased resistance if prescribed with another β-lactam antibiotic. Active against SA, HI and PsA, and also used in BCC infections.

- **Colistin**
  - *Dose*: Child 25,000 units/kg 8hrly IV
    Adult 2,000,000 (2 MU) units 8hrly IV
  - *Type*: Polymixin (binds to LPS in gram negative bacteria and disrupts cell membrane)
  - *Side effects*: Neurotoxicity: sensory and visual disturbances, vasomotor instability, confusion. Do not use with aminoglycosides
  - *Spectrum of action*: Active against PsA and other gram-negative organisms. No action against gram positive bacteria or BCC.
- **Tobramycin**
  - *Dose*: Children and adults 10mg/kg/d in 3 divided doses IV
  - *Administration*: Do not mix other antibiotics in same syringe.
  - *Type*: Aminoglycoside (binds ribosomes and prevents mRNA translation)
  - *Side effects*: Nephrotoxicity and ototoxicity. Ensure adequate hydration, and reduce dose in renal impairment
  - Monitor blood levels immediately before and 1hr after the third dose, weekly thereafter if satisfactory. Target levels are
    —Trough <1mg/L
    —Peak 8–12mg/L
  - *Spectrum of action*: Synergistic with β-lactams. Active against PsA, and preferred to gentamicin because of superior bactericidal activity and toxicity profile.

5.4.4 Exacerbations caused by B.cepacia

This should always be discussed with a specialist microbiologist. BCC are intrinsically resistant to β-lactam antibiotics, aminoglycosides and colisitin. Treatment requires combination therapy, usually including meropenem (see Chapter 3)

Antibiotics that have been used to treat cepacia include:

- Meropenem
- Imipenem
- Chloramphenicol
- Co-trimoxazole
- Doxycycline
- Piperacillin/tazobactam
- Ceftazidime
- Temocillin.

5.4.5 Pregnancy and antibiotics

Lung function can deteriorate during pregnancy (see Chapter 11), and several courses of IV antibiotics may be required.

- Antibiotics generally considered safe in pregnancy include: β-lactams (penicillins, cephalosporins) and oral erythromycin and clindamycin
- Antibiotics that should not be used include ciprofloxacin, chloramphenicol, metronidazole and IV colistin
- Aminoglycosides are probably safe, but levels need close and careful monitoring. Potential for ototoxicity is greatest in the second trimester, and may occur in the foetus independent of signs of toxicity in the mother.

5.5 **Non-antibiotic treatments**

5.5.1 **Physiotherapy**

Physiotherapy is used to assist expectoration during an exacerbation. It is widely applied, and has been shown to improve sputum clearance, though there are no controlled clinical trials on its long term benefits. No specific method of airway clearance has been shown to be superior to any other (see Chapter 4), and the choice is one of patient and physiotherapist preference. If the patient is systemically unwell, they may be less able to achieve effective cough and airway clearance, and may benefit from use of an oscillating resistance device (e.g. Flutter) or positive expiratory pressure delivered via a mask. In patients with more advanced lung disease, vigorous chest physiotherapy may be associated with desaturation during or shortly after therapy. SpO_2 should therefore be monitored and supplemental oxygen provided if necessary.

Recommendations:

- All patients with an exacerbation should be reviewed early on by a specialist respiratory physiotherapist, and airway clearance assessed. This includes patients considered for HIVT
- Patients may need additional input or devices to assist expectoration when unwell
- SpO_2 should be monitored in those with moderate-severe lung disease
- Admission affords a good opportunity to educate and reinforce physiotherapy regimes, and should be provided at least twice per day.

5.5.2 **Nutrition**

CF patients will often lose weight during an exacerbation, both because of the increased energy demands of the inflammatory response, and because of reduced appetite. Weight loss is one of the signs of an exacerbation, particularly in children and teenagers.

Recommendations:

- Patients should be weighed at start and end of treatment
- Patients admitted for an exacerbation should have an early review by a specialist dietician
- High calorie supplements should be provided to patients with poor nutrition or anorexia.

5.5.3 Management of diabetes

Poor glycaemic control, often more apparent during times of systemic illness, results in protein catabolism and weight loss. Insulin requirements usually rise during exacerbations, even if intake is reduced. Patients with impaired glucose tolerance (IGT) who do not normally require insulin may decompensate when unwell, and require the introduction of insulin. Even patients with normal glucose tolerance may have significantly elevated blood glucose (BG) when unwell.

Recommendations:

- Blood glucose should be measured in all patients on admission. Consider glucose profile for first 24 hours (i.e. capillary BG before and after meals and 1–2 times overnight)
- With young children, glucose should be checked every time bloods are taken for other assays
- If BG>6mmol/L, known CFRD or IGT, check capillary BG before and after all meals
- Patients on enteral feeds should have capillary BG measured at start, end and at least once during each feed
- Consider starting insulin if BG persistently elevated at any time of day.

5.5.4 Bronchodilators

Many patients with CF exacerbations also have airway hyper-responsiveness, and an improvement in lung function in hospitalized patients has been shown with regular nebulized salbutamol. Many patients will already be using nebulized or inhaled bronchodilators before physiotherapy, and these should be continued. Patients with known airway hyper-responsiveness or documented wheeze may also benefit from starting these treatments during an exacerbation.

5.5.5 Nebulized saline

Nebulized hypertonic saline (6%) has been shown to improve sputum clearance during an exacerbation. However, it can also cause bronchospasm and other adverse reactions in around 10% patients and should therefore be preceded by inhaled or nebulized bronchodilator. A more tolerable alternative may be 3% or 0.9% (normal) saline, nebulized before physiotherapy, to loosen secretions. These therapies can be trialled on an individual basis if patients are experiencing difficulties with airway clearance.

5.5.6 **Oral corticosteroids**

Addition of steroids during exacerbation has not been shown to improve clinical or lung function outcomes in a small study, but is associated with hyperglycaemia. The use of corticosteroids is not recommended.

5.6 **Antibiotic desensitization**

5.6.1 **Drug allergy**

Antibiotic hypersensitivity is common in CF because of the repeated high doses and long courses employed. This may place severe limitations on treatment options available to some patients. Most of the antibiotics in use can result in hypersensitivity reactions, but this is most commonly reported for piperacillin (30–50%). Hypersensitivity reactions can range from IgE-mediated immediate anaphylaxis to late onset non-specific features such as rash and fever.

Key points

- Drug allergy must be clearly documented in the patient's notes
- Patients on HIVT are taught to self-inject adrenaline (e.g. from an EpiPen®), and the first dose of any treatment course is given in hospital.

5.6.2 **Desensitization**

One approach is to desensitize the patient to prevent recurrence of allergic reaction. This involves administration of a 10^6-times dilution over 20 mins, whilst under observation. This is immediately followed by six 10-fold increases in concentration until the therapeutic dose is reached. The procedure is abandoned if any dose is not tolerated. The whole process, consisting of 7 infusions, takes 2–3 hrs and must be performed as an inpatient, under continuous observation, with resuscitation facilities to hand. If the final dose is tolerated, this is continued to the end of the course. Success rate of desensitization is around 85%.

An alternative approach employed by some units is to use a fixed concentration of antibiotics in a single bag, but to gradually increase the rate of the infusate. This has the advantage that it does not require multiple syringes to be prepared.

> ### Key points
> - Desensitization must be repeated for each course of antibiotics or if more than 1 day's doses are omitted
> - Adrenaline, hydrocortisone and an antihistamine should be readily available, with the appropriate doses for the patient calculated before starting.

Box 5.2 Example of a desensitization regimen for adults

All doses are diluted in 50ml 0.9% sodium chloride, given IV over 20 mins. If no adverse reaction occurs, the subsequent dose follows immediately.
- Ceftazidime 0.002mg
- Ceftazidime 0.02mg
- Ceftazidime 0.2mg
- Ceftazidime 2mg
- Ceftazidime 20mg
- Ceftazidime 200mg
- Ceftazidime 2000mg.

References

Breen L., Aswani N. (2008) Elective versus symptomatic intravenous antibiotic therapy for cystic fibrosis. *Cochrane Database Syst. Rev.* **3**: CD002767.

CF Trust (2009) *Antibiotic treatment for cystic fibrosis.* CF Trust, Bromley, UK.

CF Trust (2004) *Management of cystic fibrosis related diabetes mellitus.* CF Trust, Bromley, UK.

Ferkol T., Rosenfeld M., Milla CF. (2006) Cystic fibrosis pulmonary exacerbations. *J. Pediatr.* **148**: 259–64 .

Fernandes B.N., Plummer A., Wildman M. (2008) Duration of intravenous antibiotic therapy in people with cystic fibrosis. *Cochrane Database Syst. Rev.* **3**: CD006682.

Gibson R.L., Burns J.L., Ramsey B.W. (2003) Pathophysiology and management of pulmonary infections in cystic fibrosis. *Am. J. Respir. Crit. Care Med.* **168**: 918–51.

Munck A., Malbezin S., Bloch J., et al., (2004) Follow-up of 452 TIVADs in cystic fibrosis patients. *Eur. Respir. J.,* **23**: 430–4.

Parmar J.S., Nasser S. (2005) Antibiotic allergy in cystic fibrosis. *Thorax* **60**: 517–20.

Waters V., Ratjen F. (2008) Combination antimicrobial susceptibility testing for acute exacerbations in chronic infection of Pseudomonas aeruginosa in cystic fibrosis. *Cochrane Database Syst. Rev.* **3**: CD006961.

Chapter 6

Gastrointestinal disease and nutrition

Christopher Taylor and Sally Connolly

Key points

- Lung function and survival correlate with nutritional status
- 85% of CF patients are pancreatic insufficient, requiring enzyme supplementation
- Pancreatic enzyme replacement dosage should not exceed 10,000 lipase units/kg body weight
- Gastro-oesophageal reflux is common and may present with increasing respiratory disease
- Around 10% develop cirrhosis, treated initially with ursodeoxycholic acid
- Poor weight gain should prompt a dietary review. Supplementation may be required with NG or PEG feeding.

6.1 Introduction

Although progressive respiratory failure is the major cause of death, CF is a multi-system disease with important consequences for the liver and bowel. Gastrointestinal disease is the earliest clinical manifestation of CF, and may present antenatally with hyper-echoic or dilated foetal bowel on sonography. The first clear detailed clinical and pathological description of CF, in 1938, was of 49 patients with neonatal intestinal obstruction, intestinal and respiratory complications. CF was originally considered as part of the 'coeliac syndrome', since both may present with malabsorption (Figure 6.1). Prior to the development of the sweat test and intestinal biopsy, establishing a diagnosis on clinical grounds was far from easy.

The development of effective pancreatic extracts, and the demonstration by the Toronto clinic in the 1970s that aggressive management of nutritional failure improved survival, was a significant

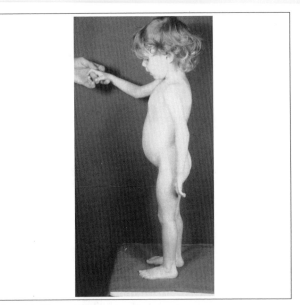

Figure 6.1 CF presenting as malabsorption

advance. These days, the importance of good nutrition and optimization of BMI, are well recognized, and respiratory complications have eclipsed gastrointestinal complications as the primary cause of mortality. Underweight patients have poorer clinical outcomes, and low weight (BMI<17 in adults, or low percent weight-for-height in children) is considered a contra-indication to listing for lung transplantation.

Gastrointestinal involvement in cystic fibrosis extends from mouth to anus. In addition to the gastrointestinal complications described below, dental enamel mineral abnormalities are also more common in CF children.

6.2 **Intestinal obstruction**

6.2.1 **Physiology**

The cells (enterocytes) which line the intestinal tract have a primary role in the absorption of nutrients, electrolytes, and water. Enterocytes, however, also secrete electrolytes and water into the gut lumen. This secretion maintains the fluidity of the intestinal contents and provides Na^+ for Na^+-dependent nutrient absorption. The secretory process involves Cl^- secretion via apical chloride channels, coupled with an inhibition of Na⁺ and water movement into the cell. Anion movement into the gut causes Na⁺ to move into the lumen via a paracellular pathway, with water following osmotically.

In the CF intestine there is a failure of CFTR-mediated Cl⁻ secretion, coupled with enhanced Na⁺ and Na⁺-linked nutrient absorption, leading to excessive dehydration of the luminal contents. This contributes to the development of the intestinal symptoms experienced by CF patients.

6.2.2 Meconium Ileus

Meconium ileus (MI) is the earliest clinical manifestation of CF, affecting 10–20% of CF infants (see also Chapter 2). Overall survival is currently over 90%.

Presentation

The condition presents within the first day or two of life with signs of intestinal obstruction (Figure 6.2):

- Abdominal distension (96%)
- Bilious vomiting (49%)
- Delayed passage of meconium (36%).

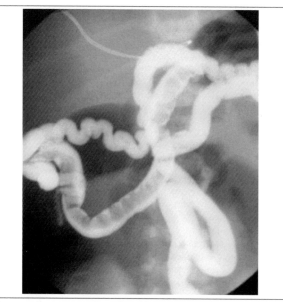

Figure 6.2 Contrast enema from infant with meconium ileus. There is a microcolon with radiolucent areas in the terminal ileum where contrast has mixed with pellets of meconium.

MI can be divided into complicated (39%–46%) and simple forms, the former depending upon the presence of associated volvulus, atresias, perforation, peritonitis and/or pseudocyst formation. Survival in complex MI is 67%, compared with 93% in uncomplicated disease. Long-term follow up suggests that survivors show similar hepato-biliary, nutritional, functional and respiratory status to non-MI CF. Despite the strong association with pancreatic exocrine insufficiency, MI is also seen in the absence of CF and occurs in pancreatic suffi-cient individuals with CF.

Investigations

Plain abdominal X-ray typically shows dilated intestinal loops and may also show a 'ground glass' appearance, representing small air bubbles mixed with meconium. Contrast enema may show micro-colon with obstruction in the terminal ileum, as in Figure 6.2.

Management

In uncomplicated cases, barium enema (Gastrografin® or Omni-paque®) plus N-acetylcysteine, combined with IV rehydration, may be sufficient to relieve obstruction. Perforation, volvulus, atresia or failed medical therapy require laporotomy.

6.2.3 Gastro-oesophageal reflux disease (GORD)

Incidence

An increased prevalence of gastro-oesophageal reflux has been reported in infants, children, and adults with CF. Based on a frac-tional reflux time >10% with an oesophageal pH <4.0, almost 20% of CF infants <6 months of age will have GORD. However, the normal range for the reflux index during the first 12 months of life includes 10%, the 95th percentile decreasing from 13% at birth to 8% at 12 months. Incidence figures for reflux in older children with CF vary between 25% and 100%, depending on patient selection. Similar high rates have been reported in CF adolescents and adults with sugges-tive symptomatology.

Effect on lungs

GORD may adversely affect lung disease by aspiration and reflex bronchospasm. Impedance-pH monitoring, combined with bron-choalveolar lavage for bile acids, has shown that both acid (pH<4) and weakly acid (pH 4–7) reflux are common in CF even in the absence of typical reflux symptoms. Oesophageal manometry has also demonstrated that GORD is not secondary to cough, but that cough follows reflux episodes.

Fundoplication

The outcome following fundoplication in children with CF is similar to that reported in large series in children without CF. There is a high rate of recurrent GORD (48%) and little apparent benefit for either nutritional or pulmonary outcomes, although children who had an FEV_1 of less than 60% predicted at the time of fundoplication exhibited an improvement in FEV_1 decline post intervention.

Management

Symptomatic reflux, or in patients in whom there is a clinical suspicion in the absence of definite symptoms, require proton pump inhibitors (e.g. omeprazole 20mg 1–2 x daily in adults). Motility agents have also been used (e.g. domperidone 10mg up to 8hrly in adults).

6.2.4 Distal intestinal obstruction syndrome (DIOS)

Presentation

DIOS, previously known as meconium ileus equivalent, occurs predominantly in patients over 15 years of age and presents either acutely, with signs of abdominal obstruction, or more commonly sub-acutely, with cramping abdominal pain and relative constipation.

Conditions that lead to dehydration may precipitate DIOS and should be avoided.

Diagnosis

The diagnosis is usually made on clinical grounds and can be confirmed with a plain abdominal film if there is clinical doubt: this characteristically shows a speckled faecal gas pattern in the right lower quadrant. Clinical examination may reveal a (tender) mass in the right iliac fossa. Volvulus may rarely occur.

Differential diagnosis

- Appendicitis
- Appendix abscess
- Mucocoele of the appendix
- Constipation
- Intussusception
- Fibrosing colonopathy
- Crohn's disease.

Treatment

- Optimize pancreatic enzyme supplementation to control steatorrhoea
- Avoid dehydration and drugs that may inhibit gut motility
- Initial treatment is polyethelene glycol (Movicol®), 20–40ml/kg/h, up to a max of 1L/h in 8 hours. Alternative preparations including Citramag® and KleanPrep® may also be used.
- Gastrografin® (diatrizoate) orally or rectally (oral, <6 years, 50ml in 150ml of water; >6 years 100ml in 400ml water: dose can be repeated after 4 hours if there is no response). Patients should take at least as much water by mouth as the volume of Gastrografin®.
- Intravenous rehydration if patient is dehydrated or vomiting.

6.2.5 Diseases of the appendix

Appendiceal disease is often mis-diagnosed as DIOS and should be considered in any patient with a right lower quadrant mass. Complications, including perforation and abscess formation, are increased—reflecting delay in diagnosis.

In CF, the appendix is frequently abnormal on ultrasound with scans showing either mucoid appendix (16%), or a pathologically thickened appendiceal wall.

6.2.6 Constipation

Constipation is common in CF at all ages: more than 70% of CF patients over 30 years of age have signs and symptoms of constipation. Small bowel and colonic transit is prolonged; studies suggest a mouth to anus transit of between 25 and 55 hours, versus a normal range of 12–48 hours.

6.2.7 Rectal prolapse

Protrusion of the rectal mucous membrane through the anus is commonly seen in association with diarrhoeal diseases and constipation. It should always be considered as a presenting sign of CF (10–13%). Rectal prolapse is rare after 4 years of age.

6.2.8 Fibrosing colonopathy

Fibrosing colonopathy is a rare condition seen almost exclusively in children with CF. It chiefly affects the caecum and ascending colon. Fibrosing colonopathy is characterized by submucosal fibrosis, with thickening of the muscularis propria leading to stricture formation. The disorder is associated with the use of high dose pancreatic enzyme supplementation (>10 000U lipase/kg/day). Evidence that the methacrylic acid copolymer enteric coating of some enzymes preparations predisposed to colonopathy needs confirmation.

6.2.9 Pancreatitis

All patients with CF have abnormal pancreatic function, however patients with mild disease (15–20%) may have sufficient pancreatic enzyme production to prevent overt steatorrhoea and promote normal weight gain. Pancreatic sufficient patients are more susceptible to episodes of pancreatitis, which can lead to progressive loss of pancreatic function and eventual pancreatic insufficiency. Pancreatitis is managed as in non-CF patients, with analgesia, fasting and IV rehydration. Abdominal ultrasound should be performed to rule out gallstones or other obstructing lesion.

6.2.10 Malignancy

Whilst there is no overall increased risk of cancer, CF patients have a significantly increased predisposition to digestive tract malignancy, around 6.5 times that of age matched non-CF population.

Tumours have been identified in the oesophagus, stomach, small and large intestine and biliary tract. Pancreatic cancer may also be found in association with cystic fibrosis, although the risk appears to relate to inherited pancreatic cancers, which represent approximately 5–10% of all pancreatic cancers.

6.2.11 **CF and other enteropathies**

Although steatorrhoea and azotorrhoea (excessive discharge of proteins in stool) principally reflect pancreatic exocrine failure, absorption may also be compromised by associated intolerances and enteropathies. Coeliac disease has been reported in association with CF, as have other enteropathies including cow's milk protein intolerance, lactose intolerance and Crohn's disease.

6.3 **Nutrition**

6.3.1 **Pathophysiology of malabsorption**

The pancreas is part of a complex digestive system including liver, gallbladder and intestinal secretions. Digestive enzymes are produced in the glandular cells (acini), stored in secretory vesicles (zymogens), and released into the proximal duodenum mixed with large volumes of bicarbonate-rich fluid secreted by the pancreatic duct cells. Each day, 6–20g of digestive enzymes are secreted into the duodenum in 2.5L of bicarbonate-rich fluid.

Enzyme secretion occurs in response to food in the proximal duodenum and is regulated by hormonal and neural interactions, involving regulatory peptides and neurotransmitters from the gut, the pancreas and the vagus nerve including secretin, CCK, neurotensin, motilin and PYY. Proteolytic enzymes are secreted as pro-enzymes which are activated by enterokinases.

In CF, pancreatic secretions are reduced, with low volumes of fluid and bicarbonate. This causes duct obstruction, and retention and activation of secreted pro-enzymes in the pancreatic ducts, resulting in destruction and fibrosis of the pancreas itself. This process begins in utero and continues after birth, leading to functional exocrine pancreatic insufficiency (PI) in the majority of CF infants. Mild mutations in the CFTR gene such as R117H and A455E, however, are associated with sufficient pancreatic function to prevent overt steatorrhoea (fatty stool; frequently floating, foul smelling and pale coloured due to the presence of undigested lipid), but may have a degree of malabsorption, particularly of fat soluble vitamins.

Enzymes are activated on reaching the intestine but require an optimum pH >5.5. The pH in the proximal intestine is usually between 5.5 and 6.5, but failure of pancreatic bicarbonate production in CF means that stomach acid entering the duodenum is inadequately neutralized. The pH in the CF duodenum is therefore often much lower than 5.0, inhibiting enzyme activity. If the pH falls further (to less than 4.0) any enzyme, either produced by the pancreas or taken in the form of pancreatic enzyme replacment therapy, will be degraded and food will not be digested.

Faecal elastase 1 is a reliable marker of exocrine PI and can be used to monitor pancreatic function over time.

Approximately 60% of CF newborns are already pancreatic insufficient, and the majority of those who will become so are pancreatic insufficient by the end of their first year. Malabsorption is, however, not simply the result of defective enzyme secretion alone but results from five separate but interdependent processes:

- Pancreatic insufficiency
- Inactivation of enzymes by pepsin and hyperacidity in upper intestine
- Failure of CFTR-mediated intestinal HCO_3^- secretion
- Deranged bile acid function
- Defective fat absorption.

6.3.2 Bile acid dysfunction

In the intestine, bile acids are secreted into the lumen of the duodenum where they contribute to the processing of dietary fat. They also activate secretory processes in the intestine. Bile acids are conserved by active reabsorption via a Na^+-dependent mechanism localized to the enterocytes in the terminal ileum. From here, they enter the portal circulation and are returned to the liver for re-secretion into the bile. This enterohepatic circulation of bile acids is extremely efficient, with less than 10% escaping reabsorption and being lost in the faeces each day.

The first step in the uptake of bile acids involves a Na^+ gradient-driven co-transporter, the ileal bile acid transporter (IBAT), located on the luminal membranes of ileal enterocytes. This operates in a similar fashion to the co-transporters responsible for Na^+-linked nutrient absorption, whose activities are altered in CF.

Thus two aspects of bile acid function in the intestine, their stimulation of secretion and their active reuptake by the terminal ileum, may be affected by CF. Bile acid malabsorption is a constant finding in untreated CF. Bile acids are also bound to the undigested protein fraction of the stool, making them unavailable for reabsorption. Faecal losses of bile acids range from 24–57 mg/kg/day. This leads to depletion of the bile acid pool and impaired fat absorption. Bile acid uptake triggers a secretion of fluid into the ileum via CFTR; this is also abnormal in CF.

6.3.3 Pancreatic enzyme replacement therapy (PERT)

Pancreatic enzymes have been available since the 1930s. Early preparations were prepared from pig pancreas by alcohol extraction; they contained the 3 major enzyme groups—amylase, lipase and trypsin—

but with considerable batch to batch variation in enzyme activity. Nevertheless, they increased fat absorption from 50–60% to 75%, improved growth and normalized blood and tissue concentrations of fat-soluble vitamins. Much activity was, however, lost through the action of gastric acid and pepsin as the powders passed through the stomach. This led to the introduction of enteric coated tablets in the 1980's. They were designed to dissolve in the duodenum at pH>5. Unfortunately, many tablets were retained in the stomach, and for those that reached the duodenum, the pH was often too low to promote enzyme activity.

In 1988, Meyer and colleagues showed that 1.4mm spheres moved from the stomach at the same rate as a test meal and from this work most of our current PERT has evolved. These enteric coated microspheres and minitablets have further improved fat absorption to 85–90%.

High strength enzymes, containing 22–25,000 units lipase/capsule were introduced in the early 1990s. These preparations gave equal or better control of malabsorption with a significant reduction in capsule consumption but as individual dosages increased, clusters of patients with strictures in the large bowel began to be reported. Fibrosing colonopathy as it was later called (see above), has been shown to be related to high enzyme intakes. Better control of enzyme dosage and changes in enzyme formulation has reduced new cases of fibrosing colonopathy to very low levels.

6.3.4 **PERT dosage**

PERT is readily available in the form of enteric coated porcine pancreatic extract in strengths ranging from 5,000 to 40,000u lipase/capsule. Dose requirements vary but are in the order of 1–2000u lipase/gram dietary fat.

Enzyme activity is affected by the following:
- Gastric emptying and gut motility
- Whether taken fasted or after food
- Size/volume of meal
- Composition of meal
- Solid/liquid
- % and type of fat
- Intestinal pH
- Liver/bile acid function.

6.3.5 **Role of the dietician**

CF is a multi-system disease and best managed by a multi-disciplinary team in specialist centres. An experienced specialist dietician who understands the level of dietetic support required and has expertise in invasive nutritional support should be part of the team.

6.4 **Management of poor weight gain**

6.4.1 **Investigations**

Nutritional problems in patients with CF should not be assumed to be secondary to pancreatic insufficiency. Coeliac disease should be excluded by appropriate serologic tests and evidence of lactose intolerance and bacterial overgrowth sought, especially in infants and children who have had surgery for meconium ileus.

Investigation of on-going malabsorption in CF:

- Coeliac screen
  - Tissue transglutaminase or endomyseal antibodies
- Lactose tolerance test
- Breath H_2 test for bacterial overgrowth
- Liver function tests
  - Transaminases
  - Clotting
- Endoscopy and small intestinal biopsy
- Hepatic ultrasound scan
- Contrast meal and follow through.

6.4.2 **Management**

General measures

Nutritional status in CF has been shown to correlate with lung function and survival. Energy requirements are increased to 120–150% of those needed by healthy individuals of the same age and sex. This reflects increased energy demands of the disease and malabsorption of protein and calories, which persists despite PERT therapy. Nevertheless, good nutritional status can be achieved in most individuals by combining a high calorie, high protein diet with adequate PERT.

Deficient intake is the chief reason for growth failure in patients with CF lung disease, particularly during exacerbations when lean tissue is rapidly lost. Support with whole protein or glucose-based supplements may help maintain body mass in the short term, but in the long term oral supplements appear to give no benefits in terms of measures of body composition or lung function.

With advancing lung disease, energy expenditure rises and anorexia is common leading to energy imbalance. The following steps should be taken before embarking on invasive nutritional support:

- Optimize oral intake
- Review adequacy of PERT
- If dose >10,000 lipase units/kg body weight add PPI to enhance PERT function
- Aggressive treatment of lung infection

- Exclude and treat GORD
- Exclude CF-related diabetes mellitus.

6.4.3 **NG and PEG** feeding

Enteral tube feeding should be used if, after oral supplements, weight for height <85% in children or BMI <18.5 kg/m^2 in adults. Other indications include failure to gain weight over a 6 month period, despite oral supplementation, or inadequate weight gain in pregnancy. Nasogastric (NG) feeding is simple and can be used successfully for short-term support during respiratory exacerbations, as an episodic boost to maintain growth or as a trial prior to gastrostomy feeding. This can be left in place, or re-inserted for each feed, depending on patient preference.

Where longer term support is required, percutaneous endoscopic gastrostomy (PEG) placement should be considered. Patients with portal gastropathy may be unsuitable for PEG, and percutaneous jejunostomy is an alternative. Feeds are usually given overnight as a complement to normal food. Careful monitoring of blood glucose is necessary when feeds are first introduced, and some previously non-diabetic patients may require insulin supplementation with feeds.

PEG insertion may be perceived negatively by patients and must be carefully timed. This is especially important in advanced disease, since post operative pain can inhibit cough and mucus clearance and exacerbate lung disease. Patients should be reassured that the gastrostromy button, on the upper abdomen, is easily concealed by clothing, and both more discrete and easier to use than NG tubes.

Both polymeric (whole protein) and elemental/semi-elemental feeds can be used to support nutrition. Elemental feeds generally contain a mixture of long and medium chain triglycerides, have a higher osmolarity and lower calorie density than polymeric feeds. Polymeric feeds with PERT appear as effective as elemental feeds in promoting weight gain. An enzyme dose based on the main-meal dose is advised with the dose split 50% at the start of the feed and a further 50% given during or immediately after the feed: enzymes should not be put down the tube. It is not considered necessary to wake patients to take enzymes.

6.5 **Hepato-biliary disease**

A variety of biliary tract and hepatic complications have been reported in CF patients. They include gallbladder diseases, comprising micro-gallbladder and cholelithiasis, and bile duct abnormalities including sclerosing cholangitits and bile duct strictures. Hepatic complications include steatosis, focal biliary cirrhosis, multi-lobular cirrhosis, neonatal cholestasis and drug hepatotoxicity.

6.5.1 Incidence

Almost all cases present in the first two decades of life and may reflect the influence of modifier genes, particularly mutations in the alpha-1-antitrypsin, mannose binding lectin and glutathione-S-transferase genes, on CFTR function. Evidence of chronic liver disease is found in 25% of CF patients but less than 10% will progress to cirrhosis. Liver failure (2–3%) and variceal bleeding (1–2%) are rare. Most cases of chronic liver disease are identified by ultrasound scans carried out as part of routine follow up in patients with an established diagnosis of CF or detection of hepato-splenomegaly on clinical examination.

Evidence of portal hypertension may develop before there is enough liver damage to affect liver synthetic function. Liver function tests that assess hepatocellular function may therefore be of limited value in identifying chronic liver disease (see 6.5.4). Alternative causes of liver disease should also be considered such as viral, drug unduced or other metabolic disorders such as alpha-1-antitrypsin deficiency or Wilson's disease.

6.5.2 Pathogenesis

The characteristic hepatic lesion in CF is focal biliary cirrhosis (Figure 6.3), although fatty infiltration is also seen. In the liver, CFTR is localized to the apical membrane of the intra-hepatic bile ducts: defective chloride secretion inhibits the hydration of canalicular-produced bile, leading to plugging of intra-hepatic bile ducts. In addition, intra-hepatic biliary epithelial cells produce excessive mucus, composed of proteoglycans, which further contributes to the viscosity of CF bile. Plugging within the intra-hepatic bile ducts exposes the hepatocytes to a high concentration of potentially toxic bile acids leading to inflammation and scaring.

Risk factors
- Male gender
- Pancreatic insufficiency
- Severe CFTR mutations
- Meconium ileus.

6.5.3 Treatment

Ursodeoxycholic acid is an anti-inflammatory that also stimulates cholangiocellular calcium-dependent secretion of chloride and bicarbonate ions, thus promoting bile flow. It is widely used to treat CF liver disease, and appears to normalize liver function tests, but long-term efficacy remains uncertain. Liver transplantation has been successfully undertaken in the presence of isolated liver decompensation with maintained pulmonary function.

Portal hypertension can lead to the development of oesophageal varices. These are treated as in non-CF patients, with variceal banding or transjugular intra-hepatic portosystemic shunting (TIPPS).

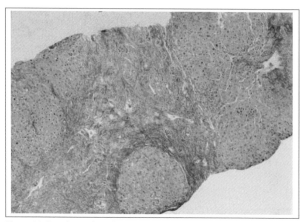

Figure 6.3 Liver biopsy (x 100) showing focal biliary cirrhosis

6.5.4 **Monitoring**

The wide variation in the reported prevalence of CF liver disease probably reflects marked under-diagnosis. CF liver disease should be actively sought as part of the annual review at least every 2 years. Often the only feature of CF related liver disease is an enlarged liver; splenomegaly if present, is a sign that the liver disease is more advanced and that portal hypertension is also present. Ultrasound should be carried out as part of the annual assessment. It is able to distinguish between normal and abnormal liver texture, the presence of steatosis, fibrosis, cirrhosis, and the presence or absence of splenomegaly. Doppler ultrasound can measure venous and arterial wave forms which provide information on blood flow, dampened or reversed flow indicating more advanced cirrhosis, and portal hypertension. Scoring systems such as the Williams/Westaby score have been devised for CF liver disease, which allow comparison between serial ultrasounds to be made.

References

Ledson M.J., Tran J., Walshaw M.J. (1998) Prevalence and mechanisms of gastro-oesophageal reflux in adult cystic fibrosis patients. *J. R. Soc. Med.* **91**: 7–9.

Littlewood J.M. (1992) Cystic fibrosis: gastrointestinal complications. *Br. Med. Bull.* **48**: 847–59.

McPartlin J.F., Dickson J.A.S., Swain V.A. (1972) Meconium ileus. Immediate and longterm survival. *Arch. Dis. Child* **47**: 207–10.

CF Trust. (2002) *Nutritional management of cystic fibrosis*. UK Cystic Fibrosis Trust Nutrition Working Group. CF Trust, Bromley, UK.

Pencharz P.B., Durie P.R. (2000) Pathogenesis of malnutrition in cystic fibrosis, and its treatment. *Clin. Nutr.* **19**: 387–94.

Smyth R.L., Walters S. (2007) Oral calorie supplements for cystic fibrosis. *Cochrane Database Syst Rev.* **24**(1): CD000406.

Westaby D. (2006) Cystic Fibrosis: Liver Disease. In: *Cystic Fibrosis in the 21st Century* (eds Bush A., Alton E.W.F.W., Davies .J.C., Griesenbach U., Jaffe A.) *Prog Respir Res.* **34**, pp.251–61. Karger, Basel, Switzerland.

Chapter 7

Cystic fibrosis related diabetes

Stephen M. P. O'Riordan and Antoinette Moran

Key points

- Diabetes is the most common co-morbidity in CF, with a prevalence of about 50% by 30 years of age
- CF related diabetes (CFRD) is generally insidious in onset, and screening with annual oral glucose tolerance testing (OGTT) is recommended
- Continuous glucose monitoring can detect abnormalities earlier than OGTT, but the clinical significance of these early changes is unknown
- CFRD is predominantly an insulin deficiency state, leading to protein catabolism, weight loss, pulmonary function decline, and early death from lung disease
- CFRD is associated with increased morbidity, some studies report a six-fold increase in mortality once CFRD is diagnosed. Clinical decline can be seen 2–6 years prior to diagnosis of diabetes
- Early intervention with insulin has been shown to reverse clinical deterioration, even in those with mild diabetes (i.e. without fasting hyperglycaemia).

7.1 Introduction

Cystic fibrosis related diabetes (CFRD) has emerged as the most common co-morbidity in persons with CF. Whilst CFRD shares features of both type 1 (T1D) and type 2 diabetes (T2D), there are important differences which necessitate a unique approach to diagnosis and management (Table 7.1). Factors specific to CF that variably affect glucose metabolism include respiratory infection and inflammation, increased energy expenditure, malnutrition, glucagon deficiency, and gastrointestinal abnormalities (malabsorption, altered gastric emptying and intestinal motility, liver disease).

Table 7.1 Comparison of different forms of diabetes			
	Type 1	Type 2	CFRD
Onset	Acute	Insidious	Insidious
Peak age of onset	Children and adolescents	Adults	18–24
Antibody (+)	YES	NO	Probably NO
Insulin secretion	Eventually absent	Decreased	Severely decreased but not absent
Insulin sensitivity	Somewhat decreased	Severely decreased	Somewhat decreased *
Treatment	Insulin	Diet, oral medications, insulin	Insulin
Microvascular complications	Yes	Yes	Yes, but less prominent
Macrovascular complications	Yes	Yes	No
Cause of death	Cardiovascular disease	Cardiovascular disease	Pulmonary disease

*Insulin sensitivity becomes severely decreased during acute illness.

7.1.2 Definitions

The American Diabetes Association (ADA) and International Society of Pediatric Adolescent Diabetes (ISPAD) place CFRD under the diagnostic heading 'Other specific types of diabetes; diseases of the exocrine pancreas'. The diagnosis is confirmed by the presence of fasting or random hyperglycaemia or a diabetic oral glucose tolerance test (OGTT) (Table 7.2). Standard OGTT categories were modified by the 1998 North American CFRD Consensus Committee to differentiate diabetes with and without fasting hyperglycaemia (Table 7.2), based on the suggestion that prognosis may differ between these two groups in CF.

CFRD falls at one end of a spectrum of progressive glucose tolerance abnormalities. Few CF patients have completely normal glucose tolerance (NGT) at all times. The earliest change is variable, intermittent post-prandial hyperglycaemia followed by impaired glucose tolerance (IGT), diabetes without fasting hyperglycaemia (CFRD FH-), and diabetes with fasting hyperglycaemia (CFRD FH+). Isolated impaired fasting glucose is rare in CF, and patients tend to maintain a normal fasting glucose level long after their post-prandial or 2-hour OGTT glucose is in the diabetic range.

There may be considerable fluctuation in glucose intolerance in a given individual with CF. Insulin resistance in CF patients is often variable, dependant on changing infectious status, medications, and nutrition. Someone with CF who has overt diabetes during an infective exacerbation may return to NGT weeks or months later.

Table 7.2 Abnormal glucose tolerance categories in CF			
Category	FPG (mmol/L)	2hr glucose (mmol/L)	Notes
Normal	<7	<7.8	
Indeterminate	<7	<7.8	Mid-OGTT glucose levels ≥11.1 mmol/L or post-prandial hyperglycemia determined by CGM in the absence of symptoms
Impaired	<7	7.8–11.1	
CFRD FH-	<7	≥11.1	Or symptoms of diabetes plus casual plasma glucose concentration ≥11.1mmol/L
CFRD FH+	≥7		
For OGTT protocol, see section 7.4.2			

7.1.3 Epidemiology

The incidence and prevalence of glucose intolerance and CFRD in patients with CF is higher than any other age-matched group. An age dependent incidence of 4–9% per year was reported in Denmark. The reported prevalence of CFRD varies depending on the screening and diagnostic criteria, and may be underestimated at centres which do not do universal screening. Whilst it can occur at any age, CFRD prevalence clearly increases as patients get older. Young age does not preclude a diagnosis of CFRD; there are isolated case reports of infants with CFRD. In the United States, 9% of 5–9 year old and 26% of 10–20 year old CF patients were reported to have CFRD (see Figure 7.1). In Denmark, 50% of patients developed CFRD by 30 years of age.

The European Epidemiologic Registry of Cystic Fibrosis (ERCF) reported 5% and 13% prevalence in age groups 10–14 and 15–19 years, respectively. A recent prospective trial from Ireland reported similar prevalence figures: NGT–69%, IGT–14% and CFRD–17% in the 10–19 years age group.

7.2 Pathophysiology

7.2.1 Genetics

CFRD mainly occurs in people with CF mutations which produce severe disease (e.g. Phe508Del) and are associated with exocrine pancreatic insufficiency. A genetic association is suggested by the increased prevalence of

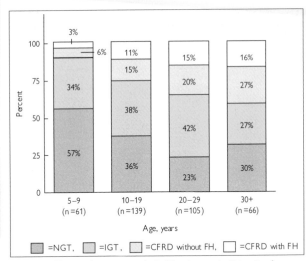

Figure 7.1 Glucose tolerance categories in CF patients at the University of Minnesota, expressed as percent prevalence within age groups. n=total number of patients studied within that age group (data from Lanng et al., 1995).

diabetes in monozygotic versus dizygotic twins. There does not appear to be a correlation with known T1D susceptibility genes such as HLA class II or insulin VNTR, but a possible link has been described between CFRD and T2D susceptibility genes associated with inflammation such as tumor necrosis factor, heat shock protein, and calpain 10.

7.2.2 **Pancreatic pathology**

Abnormal chloride channel function in CF results in thick viscous secretions causing obstructive damage to the exocrine pancreas with progressive fibrosis and fatty infiltration, Figure 7.2. This results in disruption and destruction of islet architecture leading to loss of endocrine beta, alpha and polypeptide cells. The correlation between the degree of beta-cell destruction and development of diabetes is however poor, and postmortem studies have not shown a greater loss of islets in patients with CFRD compared to those with NGT. Islet amyloid polypeptide (IAPP) deposition, which is characteristic of T2D, was found on autopsy in 69% of CF patients with CFRD, while it was absent in those without diabetes. This suggests a common pathologic mechanism between CFRD and T2D.

Beta-cell dysfunction does not appear to be related to autoimmune disease in CF. Whilst one study reported a high prevalence of DM1-associated autoantibodies in CF patients both with and without diabetes,

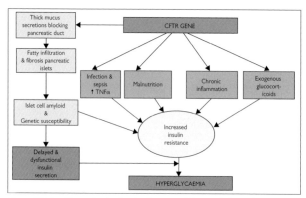

Figure 7.2 Possible mechanism for development of abnormal glucose homeostasis in CF patients, adapted from Brennan *et al.*, 2004.

these data have not been verified by other investigators. Isolated case reports of autoantibody positive individuals with CFRD suggest there may be occasional patients with co-existing T1D.

The role of insulin deficiency
The primary defect in CFRD is severe but not absolute insulin deficiency. Virtually all exocrine insufficient patients with CF, with and without diabetes, have beta-cell dysfunction. Fasting insulin and C-peptide concentrations may be normal, but there is delay and blunting of peak insulin secretion during a standard OGTT, where time to peak insulin secretion is 90–120 minutes compared to 30–60 minutes in healthy subjects. This effect is more pronounced with worsening glycaemic status. Delayed insulin secretion during the OGTT is related to loss of first phase insulin secretion, which is found even in CF patients with NGT.

The role of insulin resistance
In CF patients without diabetes, insulin sensitivity has been reported as normal or decreased. These differences are most likely related to the underlying state of health of the individual patient, since infection and inflammation influence insulin resistance. CF patients with diabetes have insulin resistance, including both decreased peripheral glucose uptake and poor insulin suppression of hepatic glucose production. Whilst insulin resistance is generally modest in CF patients who are in their baseline state of health, it can become acutely severe during infectious exacerbations. Insulin resistance is not as important as insulin deficiency in the development of CFRD.

7.3 **Survival and prognosis**

7.3.1 **Mortality in CFRD**

The presence of CFRD is associated with worse lung function, poorer nutritional status, and decreased survival compared to CF patients without diabetes. One retrospective study reported that of 448 patients with CF followed for 10 years, 25% with CFRD were alive at 30 years compared to 60% of those without CFRD. Prospective Danish data found that patients with CFRD had a median survival age of 24 years as compared to 34 years in non-diabetic CF patients. Concerning new data demonstrate a marked gender difference in survival in CFRD. Of 1,081 CF patients followed for 15 years at the University of Minnesota, median survival was 47–49 years for male and female subjects without CFRD and male subjects with CFRD; this was reduced to 31 years for female subjects with CFRD, Figure 7.3. The investigators were not able to explain this dramatic survival difference by genetic, therapeutic or clinical variables. In the UK, diabetes was associated with significantly worse lung function in women but not men with CF. It is not clear why diabetes has such a strong negative impact on women with CF.

7.3.2 **Pre-diabetic morbidity**

Several studies have shown that an insidious decline in clinical status occurs 2–6 years before the diagnosis of CFRD. In a prospective study, the decline in pulmonary function over four years was greatest in CF patients with diabetes, less in IGT, and least in patients with NGT. Pulmonary deterioration correlated with the degree of insulin deficiency at baseline. A recent study from the UK showed the decline in BMI and

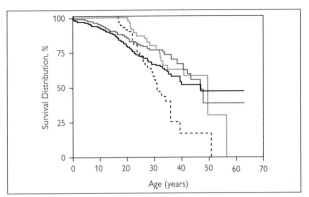

Figure 7.3 Survival curves for CF men without diabetes (blue, median survival 49.5 yrs), CF men with diabetes (grey, median survival 47.4 yrs), CF women without diabetes (black, median 47.0 yrs) and CF women with diabetes (dashed, median survival 30.7 yrs). From Milla et al., 2005.

lung function was more pronounced in those with younger onset CFRD who were twice as likely to need oral nutritional supplements and four times more likely to require enteral feeding compared to older subjects who developed diabetes. Given the known association between protein catabolism, malnutrition and death in CF, and the potent anabolic effect of insulin, the nutritional impact of insulin deficiency may be of greater consequence in CF than the metabolic impact of hyperglycaemia.

7.3.3 Complications of diabetes

Microvascular

Diabetes microvascular complications have been described in case reports and small series of CFRD patients, sometimes with significant morbidity such as blindness, glaucoma, hypertension, and renal failure. In Denmark, 36% of patients with more than 10 years duration of diabetes had retinopathy. In a larger series of 285 CFRD patients, no CFRD FH-patient (up to 14 years duration) had microvascular complications, while in CFRD FH+ complications were rare before 10 years duration of disease. However, of the 39 subjects who had CFRD FH+ of more than 10 years duration, microalbuminuria was found in 14%, retinopathy 16%, neuropathy 55% and gastropathy 50%. Whilst the prevalence of diabetes microvascular complications appears to be lower in CFRD than in other forms of diabetes, it remains important to screen for these complications.

Macrovascular

Death from atherosclerotic cardiovascular disease has never been reported in CF, despite the fact that these patients are living longer. CF patients generally have low cholesterol concentrations, although isolated hypertriglyceridemia does occur, perhaps related to inflammation.

7.4 Clinical features of CFRD

7.4.1 Presentation

The median age of CFRD diagnosis is 18–24 years, although it can present at any age. It may present at a younger age in girls. CFRD develops insidiously and patients may be asymptomatic for years. Annual routine OGTT screening is recommended for all patients ≥ 10 years not known to have CFRD.

More intensive screening (additional OGTT, blood glucose monitoring, CGM) should be considered in the following circumstances:

- Symptoms of diabetes in CF patients of all ages
  - polyuria
  - polydipsia
  - failure to gain or maintain weight despite nutritional intervention
  - poor growth velocity
  - delayed progression of puberty
  - unexplained chronic decline in pulmonary function

- During pulmonary exacerbations
- During systemic glucocorticoid therapy
- During supplemental enteral feedings
- The presence of CF liver disease
- Pre/post major surgery
- Pregnancy (ideally pre-conception, otherwise as soon as the pregnancy is detected).

Diabetic ketoacidosis can occur but is rare, mostly likely because of the persistence of endogenous insulin secretion or because glucagon secretion is also impaired. CFRD often first presents during situations where insulin resistance is increased, presumably by unmasking the underlying beta-cell defect, such as with acute pulmonary infection, chronic severe lung disease, glucocorticoid therapy, high-carbohydrate food supplementation (oral, intravenous or percutaneous gastrostomy tubes), and in association with transplantation. The incidence of CFRD is higher in those with CF liver disease.

7.4.2 Screening for CFRD

Two thirds of patients with CFRD were asymptomatic at the time of diagnosis in a prospective Danish study of 191 patients. Patients who develop overt symptoms of hyperglycaemia on presentation have a relatively greater decline in pulmonary function and weight loss compared to those identified by screening. Therefore it is important to identify patients by screening before the onset of symptoms.

HbA1c (the percentage of haemoglobin that is glycosylated, reflecting recent average blood glucose levels) has been shown by several investigators to be unreliable in the diagnosis of CFRD. Spuriously low HbA1c is hypothesized, but not proven, to be related to increased red blood cell turnover related to inflammation in patients with CF.

Whilst hyperglycemia is diagnostic for diabetes, normal fasting or random glucose concentrations do not exclude a diagnosis of diabetes.

Oral glucose tolerance test

The OGTT is the standard screening test for CFRD in much of Europe, whilst in North America measurement of fasting glucose level is more common. CFRD FH- can only be detected by OGTT. Nearly two thirds of adults with a diagnosis of CFRD do not have fasting hyperglycemia. It is important to identify these individuals because they are at high risk for both significant lung function decline and for progression to fasting hyperglycemia.

Continuous Glucose Monitoring (CGM) has the potential to identify glycaemic abnormalities earlier than the OGTT, although to date the clinical significance of this remains to be determined. CGM can highlight trends in glycaemia not previously obvious to clinicians and patients in the home environment. CGM has been recently been validated for use in children and adolescents with CF.

Table 7.3 OGTT protocol

- The patient should be clinically well at the time of testing, and not whilst taking oral steroids
- The patient is fasted from midnight before the study (8–14hrs)
- The test is performed first thing in the morning
- Time 0 blood is taken in a fluoride oxalate tube, and clearly labeled with time of testing
- A glucose load is ingested over not more than 5 minutes:
  - Adults: equivalent to 75g anhydrous glucose in a total fluid volume of 250–300ml
  - Children: 1.75g glucose per kg bodyweight, to a maximum of 75g
- Timing for the tests starts at start of ingestion
- The patient should avoid exercise or exertion during the test
- A second glucose sample is taken after 120 minutes.

7.5 Treatment of CFRD

Key points: Treatment of CFRD

- Treat CF before diabetes
- CFRD patients die from chronic inflammatory lung disease, and thus treatment of the CF takes precedence and follows the usual recommendations for this population
- As for all persons with CF, energy requirements are at least 150% of normal; with a goal of about 40% fat, 20% protein, 40% carbohydrates
- Typically these patients eat at least 3 meals and 3 snacks per day
- The insulin regimen should be adjusted to match the diet rather than asking patients to change their diet to fit an insulin regimen. This generally requires carbohydrate counting and matching insulin to carbohydrate intake
- Pancreatic supplements are essential at each meal and snack
- Modifications should be made according to the individuals needs.
- Self care education programs promote independence and encourage patients to adjust diet and insulin doses themselves
- Insulin can be delivered by multiple daily injections or through insulin pump therapy
- Monitoring with home blood glucose monitoring or continuous glucose monitoring is important
- Insulin provides an anabolic effect as well as establishing normoglycaemia.

7.5.1 **Nutritional therapy**

Malnutrition is well-known to be associated with poor growth, pubertal delay, diminished lung function and early death in CF. CF consensus guidelines stress the importance of a high calorie, high fat diet. These recommendations are the same for CF patients who develop diabetes (Table 7.4).

7.5.2 **Insulin therapy**

At present insulin is the only recommended medical therapy for CFRD (Table 7.5). Many different regimens are possible depending on individual patient needs. As in other forms of diabetes, effective basal-bolus therapy can be accomplished with an insulin pump, or with a combination of long-acting basal insulin and rapid-acting insulin to cover carbohydrates and correct hyperglycemia. Insulin therapy stabilizes lung function and improves nutritional status in patients with CFRD. There are currently no definitive data on the benefits of insulin therapy for CF patients with milder forms of abnormal glucose tolerance.

7.5.3 **Oral diabetes agents**

Oral diabetes agents are currently not recommended in CFRD. A Cochrane review identified 20 references to 14 studies, but none were randomized controlled trials. The insulin secretagogue repaglinide increased endogenous insulin concentrations but was less effective than rapid-acting

Table 7.4 Differences in the dietary management of conventional versus CF related diabetes		
	Type 1 and Type 2 diabetes	**CFRD**
Calories	≤100% of normal for age and gender—often have to watch or restrict calories to prevent overweight	Usually require 120–150% (or more) of normal caloric intake for age and gender to prevent underweight
Fat	<35% of total energy	40% of total energy
Refined sugars	Up to 10% of total energy	No restriction
Carbohydrate	45–60% total energy	45–50% of total energy
Dietary fibre	No quantitative recommendation, but encouraged due to beneficial effects	Encouraged in the well nourished, but in poorly nourished patients, it may compromise energy intake
Protein	10–20% of total energy; not >1g per kg body weight	200% of reference nutrient intake
Salt	Low intake, ≤6g /day	Increased requirement: unrestricted intake
UK CF Trust Diabetes Working Group & CF Consensus conference committee		

Table 7.5 Insulin therapy in patients with CF	
Pros	Cons
Improved well being	Increased outpatient department visits
Improved lung function	Increased complexity of daily regimen
Improved nutrition	Need for multiple insulin injections
Reduced risk of microvascular complications	and monitoring
	A second chronic illness, on top of CF
Reduced morbidity and mortality	lung disease, can be devastating

insulin at regulating post-prandial hyperglycaemia in an experimental setting. Concern has been expressed over the use of sulphonylureas in CFRD because of evidence that they bind to and inhibit CFTR, and because early experience suggested problems with hypoglycemia with these agents in CF. Agents that reduce insulin resistance are unlikely to be effective as a single therapy in CFRD, since insulin resistance is not a major aetiological factor. The gastrointestinal side effects of metformin such as nausea, diarrhoea and abdominal discomfort are unacceptable to most people with CF. Thiazolidinediones have recently been associated with osteoporosis, which calls into question the use of these drugs in CF. There are no data on the use of incretins in CF, although those that decrease gastric emptying would not be expected to be good candidates for this population.

7.5.4 Inpatient management of CFRD

During an acute illness, patients with CF are at high risk of developing hyperglycaemia. There are no specific studies of the benefits of maintaining euglycemia in hospitalized CF patients, but data from other populations have been extrapolated to suggest that intensive insulin therapy may be beneficial in this setting. Insulin requirements are often quite large during acute illness. CFRD patients who regularly receive insulin require far more, often up to four times their usual dose. It is important to remember that the insulin dose must be aggressively reduced as the patient improves. There are many CF patients whose blood glucose concentrations return to normal after illness resolves, at which time insulin therapy can be discontinued.

The primary purpose for establishing a diagnosis is to identify the expected outcome and to inform treatment decisions. ADA and WHO diabetes diagnostic criteria have changed over time to reflect new information regarding the correlation between the level of hyperglycaemia and risk of microvascular complications in T1D and T2D. Although these complications occur, they are of less concern in CFRD than the impact of diabetes on death from pulmonary disease and malnutrition. For non-diabetes abnormal glucose tolerance, there are not sufficient data at present to determine a 'cut-off' point or a particular degree of hyperglycaemia and/or insulin deficiency which confers added risk.

References

American Diabetes Association (2009) Diagnosis and Classification of Diabetes Mellitus. *Diabetes Care* **31**(1): 55–60.

Brennan A.L., Geddes D.M., Gyi K.M., Baker E.H. (2004). Clinical importance of cystic fibrosis-related diabetes. *JCF* **3**: 209–22

Dobson L., Sheldon C.D. and Hattersley A.T. (2004) Conventional measures underestimate glycaemia in cystic fibrosis patients. *Diabet. Med.* **21**: 691–6.

Finkelstein S.M., Wielinski C.L., Elliott G.R., *et al.* (1988) Diabetes mellitus associated with cystic fibrosis. *J Pediatr* **112**: 373–7.

Hardin D.S., Rice J., Rice M. and Rosenblatt R. (2009) Use of the insulin pump in treat cystic fibrosis related diabetes. *J. Cyst. Fibros.* **8**: 174–8.

Koch C., Rainisio M., Madessani U., *et al.* (2001) Presence of cystic fibrosis-related diabetes mellitus is tightly linked to poor lung function in patients with cystic fibrosis: data from the European Epidemiologic Registry of Cystic Fibrosis. *Pediatr. Pulmonol.* **32**: 343–50.

Lanng S., Hansen A., Thorsteinsson B., Nerup J. and Koch C. (1995) Glucose tolerance in patients with cystic fibrosis: five year prospective study. *BMJ* **311**: 655–9

Moran A., Hardin D., Rodman D., *et al.* (1999) Diagnosis, screening and management of cystic fibrosis related diabetes mellitus: a consensus conference report. *Diabetes Res. Clin. Pract.* **45**: 61–73.

Moran A., James P. and Carlos M. (2001) Insulin and glucose excursion following premeal insulin lispro or repaglinide in cystic fibrosis-related diabetes. *Diabetes Care* **24**: 1706.

Milla C.E., Billings J. and Moran A. (2005) Diabetes is associated with dramatically decreased survival in female but not male subjects with cystic fibrosis. *Diabetes Care* **28**: 2141–4.

O'Riordan S.M., Hill N.R., Matthews D.R., *et al.* (2009) Validation of continuous glucose monitoring in children and adolescents with cystic fibrosis – a prospective cohort study. *Diabetes Care* **32**: 1–3.

O'Riordan S.M., Robinson P.D., Donaghue K.C. and Moran A. (2008) Management of cystic fibrosis-related diabetes ISPAD Clinical Consesus Guidelines. *Pediatr. Diabetes* **9**: 338–44.

Schwarzenberg S.J., Thomas W., Olsen T.W., *et al.* (2007) Microvascular complications in cystic fibrosis-related diabetes. *Diabetes Care* **30**: 1056–61.

Chapter 8

Metabolic and musculoskeletal effects of CF

Charles Haworth

Key points

- 10–25% of adults with CF have low bone mineral density (BMD)
- Risk factors for low BMD include CFTR genotype, male gender, low body mass index (BMI), pulmonary infection/systemic inflammation, pubertal delay, hypogonadism, oral corticosteroid use, vitamin D insufficiency and vitamin K insufficiency
- Approximately 10% of adults with CF develop a non-erosive episodic arthritis characterized by painful swelling of the hands, wrists, knees and ankles
- Impaired growth in CF is associated with nutritional deficiency, lung infection and systemic inflammation.

8.1 Osteoporosis

8.1.1 Introduction

Osteoporosis is a progressive systemic skeletal disease characterized by low bone mass and microarchitectural deterioration of bone tissue, with a consequent increase in bone fragility and susceptibility to fracture. Risk factors for osteoporosis in the general population include a parental history of hip fracture, a prior history of osteoporotic fracture, low BMI, glucocorticoid use, smoking, high alcohol intake and secondary causes of osteoporosis such as rheumatoid arthritis, hypogonadism, prolonged immobility, organ transplantation, type 1 diabetes, hyperthyroidism, gastrointestinal disease, chronic liver disease and chronic obstructive pulmonary disease. The risk of fracture increases progressively with decreasing BMD. Observational (non-CF) population based studies suggest that the risk of fracture approximately doubles for each standard deviation reduction in BMD.

Dual energy x-ray absorptiometry (DXA) is the most widely endorsed methodology for measuring BMD and involves a very low effective radiation dose (<1 mSv per site). For comparison, the effective dose of a chest x-ray is 20mSv. BMD results are presented as z scores (the standard deviation score from the mean of an age and sex matched control population) or as T scores (the standard deviation score from the mean of a sex matched control population at peak bone mass).

8.1.2 Osteoporotic fractures

Fracture rates are increased in CF patients compared to the general population and most commonly affect the ribs and vertebral bodies (see Figure 8.1). These are clinically important as they are painful, prevent effective airway clearance and can lead to worsening lung infection. Rib fractures can also cause pneumothorax.

Fractures of the proximal femur (Figure 8.2) usually require surgical intervention, which is problematic in patients with advanced lung disease. A history of osteoporotic fracture may also be a relative contraindication to lung transplant listing.

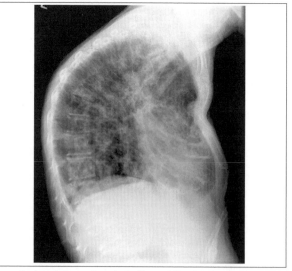

Figure 8.1 Lateral chest radiograph of a 16 year old female with cystic fibrosis and severe lung disease and osteoporotic fractures of the sternum and vertebral bodies of B6 and B7. From Latzin P, *et al.* (2005) *Thorax* **60**:616.

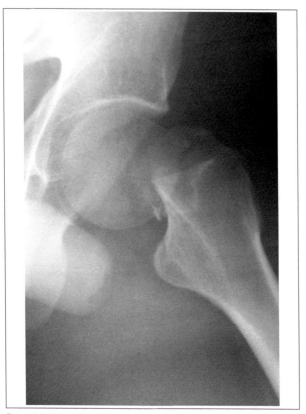

Figure 8.2 Fractured neck of femur in a 21 year old man with cystic fibrosis and osteoporosis. From Haworth CS et al. (1998) J R Soc Med. **91**(34):14–18.

8.1.3 **BMD measurements**

DXA provides an areal (2-dimensional) assessment rather than a volumetric (3-dimensional) assessment of BMD. The interpretation of areal BMD poses major challenges in healthy children due to changes in bone size related to age and puberty, and in children with chronic diseases (such as CF) in whom poor growth and delayed puberty adversely affect bone size. DXA therefore often over estimates deficits in BMD in individuals with short stature/small bones. Various corrections have been proposed such as correcting for height, pubertal stage and body composition, but these are usually only used in research settings. Consequently, BMD reference data are less reliable for paediatric, adolescent and young adult populations than adult populations.

The UK CF Trust Bone Mineralisation Working Group recommends that BMD values should be expressed as z scores in premenopausal women and in men under the age of 50 years, and as T scores thereafter. It is also recommended that the term "CF related low bone mineral density" be applied to children or adults with CF who have a BMD z score below -2, with the caveat that z scores may be unreliable in individuals of small body size.

Cross sectional studies suggest that BMD is normal or near normal in well nourished children with CF who have well preserved lung function. However, deficits in BMD are apparent in adolescents and are even more evident in young adults, such that 10–25% have low BMD (defined as having a z score < -2). Longitudinal BMD studies suggest inadequate bone mass accrual in children and adolescents with CF. In addition, young adults with CF show rates of bone loss of around 2% at the lumbar spine and proximal femur, suggesting that there may also be premature bone loss in early adult life (see Figure 8.3).

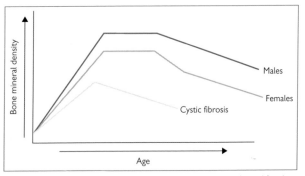

Figure 8.3 Change in bone mineral density over time in healthy males and females; and change in bone mineral density in cystic fibrosis where peak bone mass may occur early and be followed by premature bone loss.

Table 8.1 Risk factors for low BMD in cystic fibrosis

- CFTR genotype
- Male gender
- CF disease severity
  - Low forced expiratory volume in 1 second
  - Low body mass index
  - High intravenous antibiotic requirement
  - C reactive protein
  - Reduced levels of weight bearing exercise
- Pancreatic insufficiency
  - Malnutrition
  - Malabsorption of fat soluble vitamins
    - —Vitamin D insufficiency
    - —Vitamin K insufficiency
  - Calcium malabsorption
- Glucocorticoid use
- Diabetes
- Liver disease
- Pubertal delay and hypogonadism.

8.1.4 Risk factors for low BMD

The risk factors for low BMD in CF are outlined in Table 8.1.

Genotype

CFTR has recently been identified in human osteoblasts and osteo-clasts. Although the functional significance of this finding is unclear, patients with the Phe508del (ΔF508) mutation have lower BMD than patients with other genotypes, and Phe508del homozygotes have higher bone turnover than non Phe508del homozygotes, which sug-gests that CFTR may influence bone cell activity.

Gender difference

Several studies have also reported that low BMD is more common in males than females, though the cause of this association is unclear. The gender difference may reflect the protective effects of female sex hormones on BMD or relative hypogonadism in the males.

Disease severity

There is a clear association between low BMD and CF disease sever-ity. It is thought that increased expression of proinflammatory cyto-kines due to acute and chronic lung infection leads to increased osteoclast activity in CF. This is supported by the observation that biochemical markers of bone resorption are increased at the start of pulmonary exacerbations and reduce following intravenous antibiotic treatment.

Vitamin deficiencies

Vitamin D deficiency, defined as a 25-hydroxyvitamin D level <5ng/ml, is associated with osteomalacia, a condition that leads to low BMD due to an increase in the proportion of non-mineralized bone tissue. Vitamin D insufficiency, defined as a 25-hydroxyvitamin D level <30ng/ml, affects approximately 75% of patients with CF despite routine daily supplementation with 800iu ergocalciferol. Vitamin D insufficiency is associated with a relative hyperparathyroid state and induces osteoclastic bone resorption. Serum parathyroid hormone (PTH) concentrations should be measured in conjunction with 25-hydroxyvitamin D concentrations when determining vitamin D status in patients with CF. It is important to remember that 25-hydroxyvitamin D concentrations fluctuate through the seasons according to the amount of solar exposure. Thus the time of year and recent travel history should be considered when interpreting vitamin D results.

Vitamin K is an essential cofactor in the carboxylation of osteocalcin, the main non-collagenous protein in bone. In its carboxylated form osteocalcin binds to hydroxyapatite and is thought to have a role in the regulation of bone formation. Vitamin K insufficiency leads to increased levels of under-carboxylated osteocalcin, which is likely to adversely affect bone formation as it binds less effectively to hydroxyappatite. Unlike vitamins A, D and E, vitamin K is not routinely supplemented in most CF centres unless the prothrombin time is increased. As the liver is more efficient in utilizing vitamin K, a prolonged prothrombin time is a late marker of vitamin K deficiency.

Medications

Glucocorticoids suppress bone formation by osteoblasts, suppress sex steroids in men and women, and increase bone resorption in the early phase of steroid therapy. Glucocorticoids also reduce calcium absorption from the gut and increase calcium excretion in the kidney, which in turn lead to increased levels of PTH. Several studies have shown a clear association between low BMD and oral glucocorticoid use in CF.

8.1.5 Screening for low bone mineral density

The optimal age from which to start performing DXA screening for low BMD in CF is unclear. Some authorities suggest screening from about the age of 10 years, whereas others suggest performing DXA scans after peak height has been achieved to minimize the effect of bone size.

DXA scans should be repeated every 1–3 years depending on the results of the test and the clinical well being of the patient. Serial scans allow the identification of peak bone mass, following which antiresorptive treatments can be added if required. In addition, chest x-rays should routinely be examined for the presence of fragility fractures affecting the ribs and vertebral bodies.

8.1.6 Strategies to prevent low BMD

An approach to optimizing bone health is outlined in Table 8.2.

Nutrition

The CF centre dietician has a central role in optimizing bone health in children and adults with CF. Optimizing growth and lean body mass are fundamental to achieving this goal and specialist knowledge of appropriate calorific intake and pancreatic enzyme replacement therapy is required.

Vitamin supplementation

North American guidelines advocate achieving 25-hydroxyvitamin D levels of >30ng/ml, based on the finding that PTH levels rise when the 25-hydroxyvitamin D level is <30ng/ml. Achieving this level has proven extremely difficult in practice, even with high dose vitamin D replacement regimens.

Most centres prescribe between 800–1600 iu vitamin D/day to CF patients over the age of 12 years and add calcium + vitamin D supplements if the 25-hydroxyvitamin D level is inadequate (or the PTH level is elevated). As vitamin A is often combined with vitamin D in supplements, care must be taken to prevent vitamin A toxicity if dosing is increased in an attempt to boost 25-hydroxyvitamin D levels.

Calcium intake should usually be 1300-1500mg/day from the age of 8 years. Care should be taken to calculate the amount of calcium in oral supplements and overnight feeds, in addition to that taken in the regular diet.

Table 8.2 Strategies to prevent low BMD in CF

- Nutritional factors
  - Optimize growth and lean body mass
  - Optimize calcium intake
  - Correct vitamin D and vitamin K insufficiency
- Endocrine factors
  - Correct pubertal delay and hypogonadism
  - Optimize control of CF related diabetes
- Systemic inflammation
  - Optimize control of lung infection
- Encourage weight bearing exercise
- Minimize glucocorticoid use.

Vitamin K supplements are not routinely prescribed to CF patients at present, although practice is changing. Some centres prescribe AquADEK®, a CF specific multivitamin preparation that contains vitamin K, and some centres prescribe vitamin K 5–10mg daily from the age of 7 years.

Endocrine and hormonal surveillance

The UK Cystic Fibrosis Trust Bone Mineralisation Working Group recommends that pubertal development should be assessed in girls from around the age of 9 years and boys from around the age of 11 years. A morning serum testosterone should be measured annually in adult males and a menstrual history should be taken annually in adolescent/adult females to screen for hypogonadism. An endocrine referral should be made in patients with delayed puberty or hypogonadism.

Adolescents and adults should also be screened annually for the development of CF related diabetes. In patients with CFRD, blood sugar control should be optimized. Glucocorticoid treatment should be kept to a minimum.

Other therapies

An individualized exercise programme should be developed for each patient by the CF specialist physiotherapist to optimize levels of weight bearing activity.

Treatments to minimize lung infection/systemic inflammation should be implemented.

Advice, where necessary, should be provided on the adverse effects of smoking and alcohol on bone health.

8.1.7 Management of Low BMD

The standard measures outlined in Table 8.2 should be applied in all patients with low BMD.

Bisphosphonates are analogues of inorganic pyrophosphate and inhibit bone resorption. Randomized controlled trials of oral (daily and weekly regimens) and intravenous bisphosphonates show that bisphosphonate treatment leads to significant increases BMD in adults with CF. However, none of the bisphosphonate trials in CF were powered to detect changes in fracture prevalence.

Intermittent intravenous administration of bisphosphonates overcomes the poor gastrointestinal absorption and the potential oesophageal complications of oral bisphosphonates. Bisphosphonate use is associated with severe bone pain after the first 1–3 doses in a proportion of patients with CF. Pain is observed less commonly in patients starting bisphosphonate treatment after a course of intravenous antibiotics and in patients taking oral glucocorticoids, suggesting that lung infection/inflammation is a risk factor for developing bone pain. The pain tends to last up to 72 hours and can be sufficiently severe to require opiate analgesia.

The UK CF Trust Bone Mineralisation Working Group recommends that bisphosphonate treatment in adults should be considered when:

- A patient has sustained a fragility fracture
- The lumbar spine or total hip or femoral neck BMD z score is < −2 and there is evidence of significant bone loss (>4% per year) on serial DXA measurements despite implementation of the general measures to improve bone health
- A patient is starting a prolonged (greater than 3 months) course of oral glucocorticoid treatment and has a BMD z score < −1.5
- A patient is listed for or has received a solid organ transplant and has a BMD z score < −1.5.

Bisphosphonates are contraindicated in pregnancy and so females of child bearing age should be counselled before starting treatment. Bisphosphonates should also not be prescribed in patients with vitamin D insufficiency. It is usual practice to prescribe calcium + vitamin D supplements in patients prescribed bisphosphonates. Bone densitometry should be performed approximately twelve months after starting bisphosphonate treatment to assess efficacy.

8.2 Arthropathy and vasculitis

8.2.1 Arthropathy and musculoskeletal disorders

A variety of musculoskeletal problems occur in CF including episodic arthropathy, digital clubbing, hypertrophic pulmonary arthropathy and back pain. Approximately 10% of CF adults develop a non-erosive episodic arthritis, characterized by painful swelling and stiffness of the hands, wrists, knees and ankles. Symptoms usually start in adolescence and are intermittent in nature, with most episodes lasting up to a week. Anecdotal evidence suggests that symptoms are most marked during lung exacerbations and joint symptoms frequently improve with antibiotics and oral glucocorticoids. The cause of episodic arthritis is unknown but is thought to be due to immune complex formation. Very occasionally patients require treatment with long term non-steroidal anti inflammatory drugs, hydroxychloroquine or gold.

Hypertrophic pulmonary osteoarthropathy is now rare in CF and is characterized by periostitis of long bones. Symptoms are most florid during lung exacerbations and treatment is with non steroidal anti inflammatory drugs, oral glucocorticoids and antibiotics to reduce bacterial load.

Back pain and kyphosis however are common in CF and may occur in the absence of vertebral fractures. Affected individuals require assessment by a musculoskeletal physiotherapist.

8.2.2 Vasculitis

Cutaneous vasculitis is occasionally seen in patients with episodic arthropathy and is thought to relate to bacterial infection and immune complex formation. The rash is most commonly petechial and usually affects the feet and lower limbs. Erythema nodosum can also occur. Anti-neutrophil cytoplasmic antibodies against bacterial/permeability increasing–protein are often present. Treatment is with oral glucocorticoids and antibiotics to reduce bacterial load. Vasculitis can also affect the bowel, kidneys and central nervous system in CF, although this is extremely rare.

8.3 Growth

Impaired growth in CF is associated with nutritional deficiencies, lung infection and systemic inflammation. It is thought that proinflammatory cytokines such as IL-6 and TNFα reduce sensitivity to growth hormone and decrease insulin-like growth factor secretion.

Height and weight are often reduced in prepubertal children with CF and reduced height velocity is an early indicator of CF lung disease. Historical data also suggest that pubertal development is delayed in people with CF and is related to the degree of nutritional and lung function impairment. However, recent studies report normal pubertal progression as indicated by clinical pubertal staging and age at menarche, presumably reflecting improved health in childhood and adolescence.

Adult height is within the normal range for most individuals, but the mean height of adults with CF remains reduced compared to the general population.

Oral and inhaled glucocorticoids may lead to impaired growth by suppressing growth hormone secretion. Relative insulin deficiency and the development of CF related diabetes may adversely affect growth.

Growth may be enhanced by optimizing control of lung infection, optimizing nutritional parameters, treating insulin deficiency and by minimizing glucocorticoid exposure. Neonatal screening and earlier diagnosis may also lead to improved growth in CF. Recombinant human growth hormone may be used to increase height, weight, lean body mass and bone mineral content in prepubertal children with CF.

References

Aris R.M. on behalf of the Cystic Fibrosis Foundation Consensus Bone Health Group (2005) Guide to bone health and disease in cystic fibrosis. *J. Clin. Endocrinol Metab.* **90**: 1888–96.

Aris R.M., Lester G.E., Caminiti M., *et al.* (2004) Efficacy of alendronate in adults with cystic fibrosis with low bone density. *Am. J. Respir. Crit. Care Med.* **169**: 77–82.

Aris R.M., Stephens A.R., Ontjes D.A., *et al.* (2000) Adverse alterations in bone metabolism are associated with lung infection in adults with cystic fibrosis. *Am. J. Respir. Crit. Care Med.* **162**: 1674–8.

Bone Mineralisation in Cystic Fibrosis. Report of the UK Cystic Fibrosis Trust Bone Mineralisation Working Group. February 2007.

Buntain H.M., Greer R.M., Schluter P.J., *et al.* (2004) Bone mineral density in Australian children, adolescents and adults with cystic fibrosis; a controlled cross sectional study. *Thorax* **59**: 149–55.

Buntain H.M., Schluter P.J., Bell S.C., *et al.* (2006) Controlled longitudinal study of bone mass accrual in children and adolescents with cystic fibrosis. *Thorax* **61**: 146–54.

Haworth C.S., Selby P.L., Horrocks A.W., Mawer E.B., Adams J.E., Webb A.K. (2002) A prospective study of change in bone mineral density over one year in 114 adults with cystic fibrosis. *Thorax* **57**: 719–23.

Haworth C.S., Selby P.L., Webb A.K., *et al.* (2004) Inflammatory related changes in bone mineral content in adults with cystic fibrosis. *Thorax* **59**: 613–17.

Haworth C.S., Selby P.L., Webb A.K., Mawer E.B., Adams J.E., Freemont A.J. (1998) Severe bone pain after intravenous pamidronate in adult patients with cystic fibrosis. *Lancet* **352**: 1753–4.

Shead E.L., Haworth C.S., Gunn E., Bilton D., Scott M.A., Compston J.E. (2006) Osteoclastogenesis during infective exacerbations in patients with cystic fibrosis. *Am. J. Resp. Crit. Care Med.* **174**: 306–11.

Chapter 9

Psychosocial aspects of CF care

Alistair Duff and Helen Oxley

Key points

- Psychological assessment and support is essential post-diagnosis
- Behavioural difficulties are common in pre-school children. Poor mealtime behaviours are particularly problematic
- Adherence to treatment remains a significant psychosocial challenge. There is growing evidence for the effectiveness of psychological techniques and therapies for improving this
- Transition to adult CF services is a process which should involve the entire CF team and requires careful planning and execution
- Screening for emotional problems in children and their carers, and adults is essential
- Measuring health-related quality of life (HRQoL), evaluates the impact of treatments on how patients feel and function, and should routinely occur annually
- Lung transplantation can prolong life with quality for those with end-stage disease, however the psychosocial impact can be considerable
- Palliative care skills is a core-competency for adult CF team-members.

9.1 Introduction

Living with CF can be psychosocially demanding for patients and their relatives. The condition and its management impact on people's ability to respond to everyday tasks and unique life events. Whilst improved care has led to dramatic increases in median survival rates, this has been achieved by a corresponding increase in the burden of treatment, which individuals find arduous, time-consuming and intrusive. As the disease ultimately leads to respiratory failure, patients continue to potentially face prolonged periods of ill-health and reduced quality of life before death.

This chapter considers the key psychosocial challenges in contemporary clinical CF care.

9.2 **Diagnosis**

Psychological support following diagnosis is vital. As a result of newborn screening, this increasingly takes place during infancy. Whatever the child's age at diagnosis, helping parents adapt emotionally is key. This involves a combination of education and counselling.

9.2.1 **Education**

Clinicians must motivate and support parents as well as inform them. Information must be individualized and is best undertaken within the framework of an 'information exchange'.

- **Elicit**; what is already known
- **Provide**; new information/facts
- **Elicit**; understanding.

Individuals, particularly those under stress, remember only part of consultations (as little as 20%). Clinicians need to:

- Summarize key facts
- Provide written treatment plans
- Recommend reliable web-based support (see *Internet-based resources* for examples).

9.2.2 **Early intervention**

Programmes typically offer parents a combination of teaching and support, delivered to individuals, couples or groups. It is important for all CF team-members to participate.

Typical parental emotional reactions to diagnosis include:

- Intrusive thoughts and images
- Grief reactions
- Increased family strain
- Relationship difficulties and role re-evaluation.

As these sometimes develop into more intense psychological problems, 'screening' for psychosocial difficulties should take place.

Whilst contact with a CF psychologist is desirable, support and counselling can be undertaken by other suitably-qualified team members or externally, by mental health services.

9.3 **Childhood**

For many young people with CF, childhood can be a time of comparative freedom from persistent exacerbation and treatment. However, parents often worry about how CF and treatment affects their child, particularly when any behaviour problems threaten to undermine care.

9.3.1 **Feeding behaviour problems**

Mealtime behaviour problems are one of the most frequently-cited difficulties in pre-school children with CF. These are:

- Lack of appetite
- Food refusal
- Restricted food choices
- Leaving the table during mealtimes
- Crying.

This can lead to parental anxiety over calorie-intake and to parents responding differently (e.g., coaxing, force-feeding, and making different meals). In turn, these responses unintentionally reinforce the unwanted feeding behaviors. As nutrition and growth are a significant part of CF management, it is important that parents receive timely support and guidance.

Firstly, it is recommended that the Behavioral Pediatric Feeding Assessment Scale – BPFAS (Crist & Napier-Phillips, 2001), be used in clinics to identify such problems.

Secondly, effective instructions must be given to parents for minimizing feeding behaviour problems. These include:

- Having family meals
- Keeping mealtimes to no more than 20 minutes
- Give smaller portions and reward success (i.e., an empty plate)
- If necessary, have more frequent, smaller mealtimes
- Avoid coaxing, bribery and force-feeding
- Not making alternative meals.

Thirdly, advice needs to be augmented with more frequent growth-monitoring and reassurance.

9.3.2 **Procedural distress**

- Children of all ages find venepuncture one of the most frightening aspects of coming to hospital and it can result in such fear and distress that the child attempts to avoid procedures, ultimately leading to sedation or restraint (or both)
- As children with CF typically undergo many procedures involving needles during routine care (e.g., inoculations, blood tests, cannulae insertion, and port access), it is important that they learn to cope, if 'phobic' fear and compromised-care are to be avoided
- Psychological interventions are known to be effective. The key is integrating these into routine practice (see Table 9.1).

Table 9.1 The 6 'Ps'	
Prior Knowledge	• What is the child's experience of 'needles'? • What coping strategies have worked well? • Are there any technical/access difficulties? • If child is highly fearful, mark this in the notes • Avoid inexperienced practitioners attempting venepuncture
Preparation	• Prepare equipment in advance • Undertake the procedure as soon as possible in the 'consultation' • Give children information on anticipated sensations • Rehearse the procedure • Actively encourage parents to stay.
Pharmacology	• Consider topical anaesthetic options • Use conscious sedation if necessary.
Participation	• Involve the child. Let them remove plasters, and choose and clean the site • Ask if they want to watch or not • Give parents explicit instructions.
Permission to 'make a noise'	• Tell children 'it's okay to scream or cry' • Avoid telling them to 'be brave'.
Patience	• Give children the option to halt the procedure if they become frightened • Take a break • Re-introduce the procedure step-by-step.

9.3.3 Emotional difficulties

Like all children, those with CF face key psychosocial developmental tasks of developing self-esteem, confidence, and independence.

CF can interrupt these processes when children and young people 'feel different' from their peers.

Emotional problems include: anhedonia (inability to gain pleasure from enjoyable experiences), social withdrawal, sleep disturbance, worries over treatment or friendships, and physical problems made worse by worry. These can lead to clinical episodes of depression and anxiety for which there are well-established treatment protocols. As symptoms in children and adolescents can go undiagnosed it is important to increase awareness of the key features of childhood depression and anxiety and utilize widely available psychometric measures, for example:

• Children's Depression Inventory (CDI)
• Spence Children's Anxiety Scales (SACS)
• CF Questionnaire (CFQ-UK).

Starting high school is a time where children with CF are potentially emotionally vulnerable. Increasing confidence and independence at this time is crucial.

9.4 Adherence to treatment

Estimated adherence rates across all illnesses are thought to be around 50%. The aetiology of poor adherence is multi-faceted.

Treatments that are; **time-consuming**, **afford no immediate benefit** and are **intrusive**, are least likely to be adhered to. In CF these are; **physiotherapy**, **dietary recommendations** and **nebulizers**. The latter gives particular cause for concern with their prominence in respiratory drug-delivery. Usage is set to proliferate with many emerging pharmacological therapies being aerosolized.

Adolescence is the period most commonly associated with the onset of difficulties. Yet many adults also continue to struggle with the demands of care.

There are 5 general principles that CF teams need to establish to facilitate optimal adherence amongst patients:

1. Accept that partial adherence is normal
2. Establish an empathic team approach
3. Avoid blame or criticism
4. Provide written copies of treatment plans
5. Prioritize and simplify regimes, setting realistic goals.

Managing poor adherence

Interventions for improving adherence often combine several approaches; organizational, educational, motivational, and behavioural (Table 9.2).

Whilst a range of psychotherapies are effective at addressing partial-adherence, three in particular are gaining good ground: family-based interventions, motivational interviewing, and solution-focused therapy.

9.5 Transition to adult services

The importance of effective preparation and planned-transfer to adult CF services is well-recognized. Transition is not an event, but a process that involves the close working of all disciplines in the paediatric and adult CF teams (see Table 9.3).

Table 9.2 Methods to improve adherence

Approach	Exemplar
Organizational	
Shared team approach	• Develop common principles
Increase accessibility	• Outreach clinics, telephone support
Patient-friendly approach	• Simplify treatments, adapt treatments to lifestyles and minimize adverse side-effects
Provide education	
CF, treatment, side-effects	**How**—Leaflets, videos, CD-ROMs, slide-shows, handouts, demonstrations
Adherence problems in complex regimens	**Where**—During routine clinic visits, home-visits, telephone consultations
Barriers to adherence	**By whom**—Entire CF team
Improving adherence	
Relapse-prevention	
Motivational	
Express empathy	Listen to and understand patients' perspectives
Respect choice to 'change or not'	
Identify discrepancies between beliefs, behaviours and goals	Consider advantages/disadvantages of change (avoid arguing *for* change)
Clarify treatment goals and remove barriers to change	Accept that goals of treatment vary
Work *with* resistance	Never directly confront patients
Provide regular feedback	Positively-reinforce any small changes or contemplation of change
Support the development of patient self-efficacy	Develop patients' growing sense that they *can* achieve change
Behavioural	
Self-monitoring	• Patient diaries
Set achievable goals	• Write 'contracts' with patients about specific adherence behaviours required
Behavioural contracting	
Positive feedback and reinforcement	• Systematically encourage and reward.

Barriers to effective transition:

• Patients who are sick or who undergo rapid deterioration
• Fears (often unrealistic), about adult care or the transfer process (e.g., perceptions of 'moving closer to death' or increased risk of cross infection)
• Low self-esteem or self-efficacy
• Paediatric team-members becoming overly-attached.

Table 9.3 Psychosocial benchmarks for effective transition	
Paediatric Team	• Begin preparation for transition during childhood by encouraging appropriate levels of self-care, self-advocacy and participation in decision-making • Reinforce positive messages about contemporary adult life with CF where appropriate • Review progress annually • Help parents anticipate their own changing roles • Reassure parents that they will not be 'excluded' by the adult CF team if the patient wishes them to be involved • Make detailed preparation for transfer on an individual transition plan, led by a key worker who has close familial involvement.
Paediatric & Adult Teams	• Arrange meetings with adult CF team and visits to the adult centre • Use 'readiness' as an indicator of transfer rather than 'age' (up to the age-limit of the paediatric service) • Assess and document barriers to transfer and address these • Effective communication between teams and sharing detailed information is essential at transfer.
Adult Team	• Quickly establish appropriate care plans and goals based on transition information and developmental needs • Regularly update knowledge of adolescent and young adult psychosocial development.

9.6 Psychological difficulties in adulthood

Adults with CF have to deal with many stressors leading to some developing significant psychological problems that require specialist intervention. At times, many more have difficulty in coping, lowering their quality of life as a result.

9.6.1 Quality of life (QoL)

• There is increasing recognition that measuring health-related QoL (HRQoL), yields particular information about the impact of CF on patients that only they can know about

• HRQoL is an excellent way of describing and evaluating the impact of therapies on how patients feel and function. A crucial requirement of treatments should be clear demonstration of benefits

• Although there are many CF QoL measures, one that is becoming established internationally is the Cystic Fibrosis Questionnaire – CFQ (Quittner et al., 2000), incorporating 12 dimensions of CF-

QoL including: physical functioning, emotional state, social limitations, embarrassment, body image and treatment constraints
• The UK version (CFQ-UK), has recently been made widely available.

9.6.2 **Screening for specific psychological difficulties**

Early identification of patients at 'high risk' of psychological difficulties is very important. Psychological screening should therefore form part of the annual assessment for adults with CF. Specific screening tools (e.g., the Hospital Anxiety and Depression Scale – HADS), identify problems quickly. Clinical scores need to be followed-up by a CF psychologist who will consider the problems and coping difficulties in the wider context of the patient's psychological functioning.

9.6.3 **Psychopathology**

Wide-ranging psychological issues can arise in adults with CF (see Table 9.4), requiring specialist intervention; most commonly anxiety and depression which can impact negatively on treatment adherence and QoL.

9.6.4 **Psychological interventions**

Whilst little is known about the effectiveness of psychological interventions in CF specifically, the evidence-base for cognitive behaviour therapy (CBT) is strong for certain psychological problems and must be available to the CF team. Other useful psychological interventions include: motivational interviewing, systemic work, solution-focussed therapy and 'mindfulness' techniques.

Support for families of patients is also essential. This is often provided by the CF social worker, alongside other roles (e.g., providing support and advice on financial, educational, vocational, and housing issues).

Table 9.4 Common psychological problems in adults with CF

• Anxiety disorders (including panic attacks, phobias, generalized anxiety disorder and obsessive compulsive disorder)
• Depression or significant low mood (which can involve self-harm and suicidal ideation or acts)
• Post-traumatic stress reactions to medical events (e.g. haemoptysis, pneumothorax)
• Low self-esteem and confidence
• Anger
• Sleep disturbance
• Distorted body image
• Disordered eating
• Family or relationship difficulties
• Substance misuse
• Problems managing CF (including coping with increasingly invasive procedures and deteriorating health).

9.7 End of life care

Deaths occurring at comparatively young ages, after long relationships between patients, families, and teams, and where prognosis can be hard to predict, can make end-stage care particularly complex and distressing.

9.7.1 Transplantation

For patients who meet the necessary criteria, lung transplantation is perhaps the only intervention that can prolong life with quality (see Chapter 10). This increasingly happens in adult groups, but not exclusively so.

- The process of referral, listing and waiting is lengthy and more patients die waiting than ultimately undergo surgery
- Psychological stressors increase as the process unfolds, but being told of the 'need' and 'making the decision' is reported as being particularly traumatic
- Psychosocial assessment should be part of the process of referral to transplant centres, identifying:
  - QoL
  - Coping
  - Decision-making
  - Family, social and financial support
  - Potential psychosocial contra-indicators (e.g., alcohol or drug-addiction, chronic poor adherence)
- The lung transplantation process impacts on end of life care, with many patients dying in acute, intensive environments.

9.7.2 Palliative care

The goal of 'a good death' is more likely to be achieved if CF teams have the skills to address these difficult issues without avoidance.

Table 9.5 Key psychological tasks in end of life care

- Help teams discuss care-decisions with patients, who can then make informed choices and communicate these
- Ensure that patients' psychological, spiritual and existential needs are given 'air-time' and addressed
- Identify barriers to optimal palliative care
- Deliver psychological interventions for depression, anxiety, pain, and insomnia
- Discuss bereavement issues with families (and fellow-patients)
- Facilitate peer-support for team-members
- Assist in ensuring that palliative care training is met.

Patients, and where appropriate, their relatives, should receive timely information about options for end of life care, in order to make choices and decisions.

Talking about death does not make it happen sooner! It gives patients opportunities to consider what they have achieved in their lives and what they have left to do before they die.

Using the principles of palliative care is important, even if these need adapting for CF care. It gives teams opportunities to consider often under-diagnosed symptoms (e.g., pain and nausea), and psychological distress.

References

Bryon M., Buu A, Davis M.A., Watrous M., Quittner, A.L. (2009) CFQ-UK: Cystic Fibrosis Questionnaire, a health-related quality of life measure (English UK, Version 1). Forest Laboratories UK Ltd. Bexley.

Crist W., Napier-Phillips A. (2001) Mealtime behaviors of young children: a comparison of normative and clinical data. *J. Dev. Behav. Ped.* **22**: 279–86.

Duff A.J.A., Latchford G.J. (2010) Motivational interviewing adherence problems in cystic fibrosis. *Ped Pulmonol* **45**: 211–20.

Duff A.J.A., Oxley H. (2007) Psychological aspects of CF. In M., Hodson, D. Geddes, & A. Bush (Eds.) *Cystic Fibrosis* 3rd Edition, pp.433–41. London: Hodder Arnold.

Fielding D.M., Duff A.J.A. (2006) Adherence to treatment in children and adolescents living with chronic illness. In F.D. Burg, J.R. Inglelfinger, R.A. Polin, A.A. Gershon (Eds) *Gellis and Kagan's Pediatric Therapy* 18th Edition; p.229. Elsevier. New York.

Ford D., Flume P.A. (2007) Impact of lung transplantation on site of death in cystic fibrosis. *J. Cyst. Fibrosis* **6**: 391–5.

Kazak A.E., Simms S., Rourke M.T. (2002) Family systems practice in Pediatric psychology. *J. Pediatr. Psychol.* **27**: 133–44.

Kettler L.J., Sawyer S.M., Winefied H.R., Greville H.W. (2002) Determinants of adherence in adults with cystic fibrosis. *Thorax* **5**: 459–64.

Paediatric Psychology Network Position Paper (2010) Evidence-based guidelines for the management of invasive and/or distressing procedures with children. British Psychological Society. London.

Quittner A.L., Barker D.H., Snell C., *et al.* (2008) Prevalence and impact of depression in Cystic Fibrosis. *Curr. Op. Pulm. Med.* **14**: 582–8.

Quittner A.L., Sweeney S., Watrous M., *et al.* (2000) Translation and validation of a disease-specific quality of life measure for cystic fibrosis. *J. Pediatr. Psychol.* **25**: 403–14.

World Health Organization (2003) Adherence to long term therapies: evidence for action. Geneva. WHO.

Chapter 10

Lung transplantation

Laura Tanner and Andrew J. Fisher

Key points

- Lung transplantation should be considered a treatment option for severe CF lung disease uncontrolled on maximal medical therapy
- Lung transplantation is not a cure for CF and ongoing CF team care should continue after lung transplantation
- Referral to the transplant centre should be made in a timely fashion using international referral criteria as a guide
- Pre-transplant assessment of physical, functional, microbiological and psychological parameters is used to determine candidate suitability
- Pre-transplant optimization of physical functioning and nutrition is essential to increase the chance of a successful transplant outcome
- Immunosuppressive drugs are required lifelong after lung transplant and are associated with significant side effects which can themselves cause morbidity
- Early complications include primary graft dysfunction, infection and acute rejection of the transplanted lungs
- Long-term survival is limited by development of chronic graft dysfunction causing marked remodelling of the airways known as *Obliterative Bronchiolitis*.

10.1 Introduction

Lung transplantation, when successful, offers the possibility of an active and extended life to selected patients with severe end stage lung disease which is failing on maximal medical therapy.

The modern era of lung transplant started in the early 1980s. Currently approximately 2000 lung transplants are performed each year worldwide. Changes in patient selection, surgical techniques, antibiotic and immunosuppressive medication regimens have steadily improved outcomes. Today many lung transplant recipients can expect to survive in excess of 10 years.

The primary aim of lung transplantation is to improve survival with the secondary benefit of improving quality of life. Due to the shortage of donor organs, lung transplantation will rarely be performed for improvement in quality of life alone. As a result, indicators of disease severity and of an adverse prognosis must also be satisfied in candidates.

Due to the limited supply of donor organs each patient referred must be assessed for suitability and the likelihood of a successful outcome determined before being placed on the active lung transplant waiting list.

10.2 Lung transplantation for CF

Due to advances in the organisation of CF care and increasingly prompt and aggressive treatment of infections, patients with CF are surviving longer with an average survival age of 30–40 years.

CF is the third most common condition for which lung transplantation is performed, accounting for 14% of all lung transplants worldwide.

Post-transplant survival for CF is among the highest of all transplantable chronic lung conditions with an 85% 1 year survival, 70% 3 year survival and 50% 5 year survival worldwide (International Society of Heart and Lung Transplant registry data). However, centres very experienced in performing lung transplants for CF can exceed this, achieving a median survival of over 10 years.

Lung disease is the primary cause of death in 80% of CF patients meaning that lung transplantation is a treatment option required by many. Despite attempts to increase organ donation, demand significantly outstrips supply, waiting lists are growing and there remains a disappointing number of deaths among those on the waiting list.

10.2.1 Surgical approach

All CF patients require a bilateral lung transplant due to chronic bacterial and fungal colonization and the risk of re-infection of the transplanted lung from the colonized native lung.

Bilateral lung transplantation is often performed through a "clamshell" or transverse incision (see Figure 10.1). The native lungs are removed, usually with the patient on cardiopulmonary bypass, and the new lungs implanted one at a time (often referred to as a single, sequential lung transplant).

10.2.2 When to refer

Each patient has a window of opportunity when the benefits of transplantation, with regards survival and quality of life, outweigh the risks of surgery and peri-operative complications.

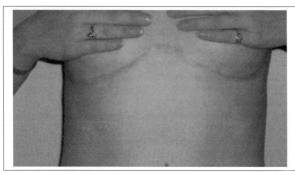

Figure 10.1 Clamshell incision on a female CF patient who has previously undergone bilateral lung transplantation.

Patients should be referred early enough to prevent them becoming too sick for transplantation if their condition deteriorates. Timely referral is paramount due to the shortage of donor organs and the risk of death on the waiting list (see Box 10.1).

Once listed for lung transplant, the waiting time can vary widely depending on blood group, size and the condition of other candidates on the waiting list. Current opinion is that a patient should be referred when their predicted 2 year survival is approximately 50%. This can be difficult to ascertain due to the heterogeneous nature of CF lung disease and as yet no accurate prognostic model for CF lung disease exists.

Most transplant centres would prefer early referral to ensure enough time for rational assessment of the patient, management of any areas of concern, optimization of the patient's pre-transplant condition and ultimately patient education to allow an unhurried and informed decision regarding lung transplantation.

Listing for transplant is required imminently in the context of:

• Oxygen dependent respiratory failure
• Hypercapnia
• Pulmonary hypertension.

10.2.3 Recipient selection

Lung transplantation carries a significant morbidity and mortality risk. To ensure the best possible outcome patients are assessed using strict selection criteria and their pre-transplant condition is optimized as best as possible.

Conditions or targets, such as weight management or physical conditioning, may be set by the transplant centre which must be achieved before transplantation is considered appropriate.

Box 10.1 **CF specific referral criteria (ISHLT guidelines)***

- FEV_1 <30% predicted or rapid decline in FEV_1 (especially if female and <18 years)
- Increasing frequency of exacerbations requiring intravenous antibiotics
- Exacerbation of pulmonary disease requiring ITU stay
- Refractory or recurrent pneumothoraces
- Recurrent haemoptysis not controlled by embolization.

* ISHLT: International Society of Heart and Lung Transplantation

Box 10.2 **Absolute contraindications to lung transplantation**

- Malignancy in last 2 years (excluding BCC and SCC of skin)
- Untreatable advanced dysfunction of additional major organ system
- Significant chest wall or spinal deformity
- Documented on-going non-compliance
- Untreatable psychiatric or psychological condition affecting ability to cooperate or comply with treatment
- Absence of reliable, consistent social support system
- Current substance addiction or use
- Acute extra-pulmonary sepsis/uncontrolled systemic infection
- Known immunosuppression drug intolerance
- Inability to adequately treat pulmonary infections*
- Colonization with Burkholderia cenocepacia genomovar III (most centres worldwide)*.

* CF specific contra-indications

10.2.4 Special considerations in CF

Lung transplantation will improve respiratory function but extra-pulmonary disease in the sinuses, intestines, pancreas and upper airways remains and can influence outcome post transplantation.

Sinus and upper airways disease

Colonization of the sinuses, upper respiratory tract and large airways with multi-resistant organisms are a potential risk for pulmonary re-infection post-transplantation. Although isolation of pre-transplant organisms after transplantation is common there is no evidence that sinus surgery and washout pre-transplant affects outcomes post-transplantation. Many transplant centres use nebulized antibiotics in an attempt to prevent clinical infection in the context of immuno-suppression.

> **Box 10.3 Relative contraindications to lung transplantation**
>
> - Age >65 years (single lung) or >60 years (bilateral lung)
> - Critical or unstable condition
> - Severely limited functional status with poor rehabilitation potential
> - Colonization with highly resistant or highly virulent organisms
> - Severe or symptomatic osteoporosis
> - Invasive mechanical ventilation
> - Co-morbidities (no end organ damage, must be optimally treated)
> - Poorly controlled extra-pulmonary CF disease manifestations*
> - Poor nutritional status: BMI<18 *
> - Liver cirrhosis with hepatic dysfunction and uncontrolled portal hypertension (potential for lung/liver transplant in selected candidates and centres)*
> - Colonization with *Mycobacterium abcessus**
> - Intra-cavitary Aspergillus situated near the pleura*
> - Severe pleural thickening*.
>
> * Contraindications specific to CF

Pneumothoraces

Management of recurrent pneumothoraces can present problems in the management of patients awaiting lung transplant. Current recommendations are to perform the minimum intervention required to control and stabilize the patient's condition. Studies suggest that patients who have undergone previous pleural procedures do not have adverse outcomes after lung transplant compared to those who did not. Blood pleurodesis has not been shown to offer any benefit over other interventions.

Respiratory infections

Improvements in peri-operative mortality in the CF population may be due to advances in microbiological testing and the use of targeted antibiotic regimens at the time of transplant.

CF patients are often chronically infected with multi or pan-resistant organisms and the risk of seeding infections to the pleura, or systemically, at the time of transplantation is considerable. Repeated antibiotic use can lead to multiple antibiotic hypersensitivities in this population, limiting the antibiotics available for use. Desensitization may need to occur pre-transplant if there are limited antibiotic options (see Chapter 5).

To reduce peri-operative infection risks to an acceptable level an antibiotic regimen must be found that adequately treats recipient organisms before transplant can be considered. Patients may not be listed for transplant until an effective combination of antibiotics can be identified.

Many centres use multiple combination synergy testing to find the best combination of antibiotics for use at the time of transplant. It is important to regularly update the transplant centre about recent infections and antibiotic use, in addition to sending regular sputum samples.

Many organisms initially thought to adversely affect transplant outcomes have not been proven to increase mortality in isolation. The risk that specific infections contribute depends on the presence of other relative contraindications.

- Multi-drug or pan-resistant *Pseudomonas aeruginosa* has not been shown to increase mortality post transplantation, and is therefore not a contraindication to transplantation
- Intracavitary *Aspergillus fumigatus* or mycetoma situated near the pleura can be seeded at the time of transplant. Aggressive and comprehensive treatment is needed but such patients have been successfully transplanted
- Atypical mycobacteria other than *Mycobacterium abcessus* are not a contraindication to transplantation as long as they have been adequately controlled.

Some organisms have been associated with an increased morbidity and mortality in some centres after lung transplantation:

- *Mycobacterium abcessus*, a rapidly growing mycobacterium, has a high risk of recurrence due to being extremely difficult to eradicate and having a propensity to infect soft tissues. Removal of the lungs does not necessarily indicate complete removal of the organism. It is associated with significantly increased morbidity and mortality and requires an individual approach to assess risk

---

Box 10.4 Organisms not associated with an increase in mortality

- Multi-drug or pan-resistant *Pseudomonas aeruginosa*
- *Staphylococcus aureus*
- Meticillin resistant *Staphylococcus aureus*
- *Stenotrophomonas maltophilia*
- *Alcaligenes xylosoxidans*
- *Aspergillus fumigatus*
- Atypical mycobacterium (excluding *Mycobacterium abcessus*).

- *Burkholderia cenocepacia* has been shown to be detrimental to survival post transplantation with a 30–40% increase in mortality (50% survival at 1 year). This degree of increased mortality acts as a contraindication to lung transplantation in most centres worldwide. Other organisms within the *Burkholderia cepacia* complex do not carry this increased risk in well selected recipients.

10.2.5 Non-pulmonary manifestations of CF and lung transplantation

Non-pulmonary manifestations of CF can have a major impact in the early post-operative period.

Pancreatic insufficiency

More than 85% of patients with CF require pancreatic enzyme supplementation due to pancreatic insufficiency. Pancreatic enzymes should be given with ciclosporin to improve absorption, as adequate levels of immunosuppressant can be difficult to achieve in CF patients.

Distal intestinal obstruction syndrome (DIOS)

Gastrointestinal complications such as abdominal pain and diarrhoea are common after lung transplantation in patients with CF. DIOS is the most significant early GI complication with a frequency of approximately 20%. Active prevention is vital with early administration of pancreatic enzymes and vigilance to enable early diagnosis and prompt treatment (see Chapter 6).

Gastro oesophageal reflux disease (GORD)

GORD is common in CF patients and can worsen after surgery due to gastroparesis and potential damage to the vagus nerve. Reflux is associated with development of chronic lung allograft dysfunction and so needs to be treated promptly and aggressively, with fundoplication if necessary.

Liver disease

Liver disease occurs in one third of patients with CF and is a major complication that is becoming more relevant as extra-hepatic disease is more effectively treated. Patients with advanced liver disease undergoing lung transplantation have a high morbidity and mortality resulting from post-operative hepatic insufficiency. A combined liver-lung transplant may be considered for those patients with end stage pulmonary disease and progressive advanced liver disease.

Nutrition

Most transplant centres will not consider transplantation if BMI is <18, as poor nutrition is associated with poor outcomes post transplantation. Often overnight nasogastric tube feeding or placement of a percutaneous gastrostomy tube is recommended to maintain a safe weight (see Chapter 6). A minimum weight may be stipulated at assessment and even once listed the patient may not be transplanted if below this target weight.

Diabetes mellitus

CF related diabetes occurs in 30% of adult patients. Good glycaemic control is important as uncontrolled diabetes can adversely affect outcomes such as surgical healing and prolonged infection in the post-operative period (see Chapter 7). Good control of CF related diabetes helps to maintain weight in the pre-transplant period. 20% of patients develop diabetes after transplantation due to a combination of calcineurin inhibitors and high dose steroids.

Osteoporosis

Osteopenia is common in the CF population and should be considered for treatment with bisphosphonates and calcium and vitamin D supplementation before transplantation (see Chapter 8). Bone mineral density will be further reduced post transplantation by long term steroid and immunosuppressant use.

Other considerations

Mechanical ventilation is considered a relative contraindication to transplantation in most transplant centres. In the general population invasive ventilation is a risk factor for post-transplant mortality but some studies suggest this is not the case in CF. There is no consensus between transplant centres but if the patient has been assessed and listed before intubation and there is a short ventilation time they may be successfully transplanted.

Chronic *Clostridium difficile* carriage occurs in many CF patients and can cause infection in the early post transplant period due to aggressive use of antibiotics and immunosuppression. Presentation is often atypical with an absence of diarrhoea. Complications include toxic megacolon and fibrosing colonopathy, frequently requiring surgery and associated with a high mortality.

10.3 The process of lung transplantation

10.3.1 Pre-transplant

Patients will undergo a 3 or 4 day assessment process with numerous investigations performed to assess disease severity, suitability for transplant and highlight areas for medical optimization, as well as ability to cope psychologically with transplantation issues.

Transplantation is a major life event and is a huge emotional, financial and physical ordeal for the candidate and their carers. For this reason it is essential that a robust support system exists. Carers should be prepared to stay with the candidate at the hospital at the time of transplant and provide support during the peri-operative recovery period.

The patient is committing to a lifetime of immunosuppressive medication and susceptibility to infection. Compliance with medication, minimizing infection risk, following post transplant management advice and lifestyle advice is essential for a successful outcome.

To minimize organ ischaemic time patients are often notified to come to the transplant centre whilst the potential donor lungs are still being assessed. This might lead to the potential transplant being cancelled and may happen a number of times before a candidate is successfully transplanted.

10.3.2 **Recipient and donor matching**

Matching of a recipient to donor organs is done by blood group and predicted total lung capacity (TLC) using height, age and sex. Predicted recipient TLC is matched to predicted donor TLC to match for size. The severity of illness is considered but time on the list is not a prioritization indicator for transplantation. Race and gender have no bearing on matching.

10.3.3 **Post-transplant complications**

Complications post lung transplantation can be divided into early (<6 months) and late (>6 months) (Table 10.1 and 10.2). Shared care between the transplant centre and local CF centre is encouraged to ensure continued management of non-pulmonary CF related disease.

Acute rejection

Acute rejection is common, occurring in up to 50% of patients in the first 6 months. To allow early detection and prompt treatment some transplant centres perform regular, surveillance bronchoscopy and transbronchial biopsy during the first year after transplantation. Acute rejection is often asymptomatic or can present insidiously and non-specifically. Symptoms include low-grade fever, lethargy, dyspnoea and small pleural effusions on CXR. There may be an associated fall in pulmonary function. If acute rejection is suspected referral to the transplant centre for consideration of transbronchial biopsy and prompt treatment with augmented immunosuppression is required.

Malignancy

The incidence of malignancy is increased after lung transplantation due to the effects of the immunosuppressants on immune function. Although there is an increased incidence of solid organ tumours, the commonest malignancy after transplantation is skin cancer and patients must therefore use high factor sun block.

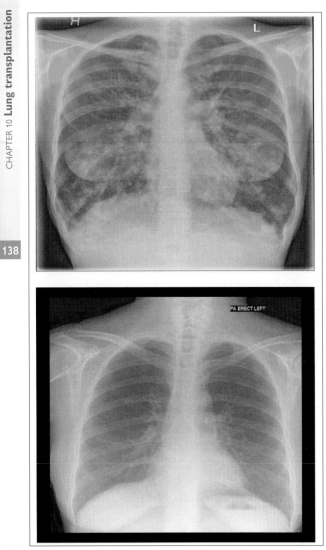

Figure 10.2 CXR of a CF patient pre- and post-transplantation

Post transplant lymphoproliferative disorder (PTLD)

PTLD is the second commonest malignancy after skin cancer in solid organ transplant recipients. After lung transplantation the incidence is 4–10%, and in the majority of cases it is driven by Epstein-Barr virus (EBV) infection. PTLD can occur in any organ including the lung, intestine, liver, and central nervous system. The commonest presenting features are fever and lymphadenopathy, followed by symptoms caused by extranodal involvement. Asymptomatic nodules in the lung or liver can be the first sign of the condition. Diagnosis requires excisional biopsy to provide tissue for histology and evaluation of EBV status. A reduction in the level of immunosuppression may be effective in some individuals but those who fail to respond to this approach may require chemotherapy.

Bronchiolitis obliterans syndrome (BOS)

Long-term survival after lung transplantation is limited by the development of a progressive dysfunction of the transplanted lungs, which is often labelled as 'chronic rejection'. The pathological changes are classified as an obliterative bronchiolitis resulting from chronic inflammation and fibrotic repair of small and medium sized airways causing luminal obstruction. Clinically this manifests as progressive airflow obstruction which, in the absence of other identifiable causes of graft dysfunction, is termed bronchiolitis obliterans syndrome (BOS). BOS affects 50–60% of patients surviving more than 5 years after lung transplant and has a three year mortality >50%. Clinically patients present with dyspnoea, cough, chest tightness and reducing exercise capacity and the condition is often accompanied by increased bacterial infections.

Presentation with BOS can be insidious or acute with a variable rate of progression, which is impossible to predict at the outset. Possible presentations include:

- Sudden onset with rapid decline in lung function
- Insidious onset with slow, progressive decline over time
- Initial rapid decline in FEV_1 followed by a prolonged period of stability.

A high index of suspicion, regular surveillance of lung function by spirometry and prompt contact with transplant centres remain vital to early detection of BOS. BOS should be suspected in patients with an irreversible reduction in pulmonary function to <80% best post-transplant FEV_1 in whom infection and acute rejection have been excluded.

- Recurrent episodes of acute rejection
- Lymphocytic bronchitis/bronchiolitis
- Pseudomonas infections
- HLA mismatching
- CMV pneumonitis
- Gastro-oesophageal reflux (GORD)
- Community acquired respiratory virus infection
- Medical non-compliance.

10.3.4 Infections after transplantation

The risk of infection is higher after lung transplant than after other solid organ transplants. This is due to the higher immunosuppression levels required, exposure of the lung allograft to the external environment and denervation causing impaired cough and mucociliary clearance.

Viral infections

Cytomegalovirus (CMV) is the commonest viral pathogen isolated in lung transplant recipients. CMV IgG negative recipients in receipt of a lung from a CMV IgG positive donor are at the highest risk of developing significant invasive disease.

The incidence of significant invasive disease has been significantly reduced by the use of prophylactic anti-viral strategies in CMV donor-recipient mismatches. Presentation of CMV disease can be acute, with a sudden onset of symptoms, or insidious with low-grade temperatures, lethargy and malaise.

CMV disease can affect any organ but most commonly affects the lung and/or the GI tract, presenting with dyspnoea and/or abdominal pain and diarrhoea. Diagnosis is suspected clinically and confirmed by a significant elevation in viral DNA copies using CMV PCR or demonstration of CMV viral inclusion bodies in lung or gut biopsy.

Community-acquired respiratory viral infections are more common in lung transplant recipients and may cause acute loss of lung function. Seasonal influenza vaccination is recommended for all lung transplant recipients. Infections with such viruses have been associated with the development of bronchiolitis obliterans syndrome.

Bacterial infections

Bacterial infections can occur anytime after lung transplantation. Infection of the transplanted lungs with Pseudomonas species is common in CF recipients and is often treated with regular nebulized antibiotics to reduce the risk of ongoing airway injury. Typical respiratory bacterial pathogens are more likely to be the cause of acute bacterial respiratory infections than rarer opportunistic bacteria.

Fungal infections

Candida and Aspergillus species account for the vast majority of significant fungal infections. Colonization is frequent with a combined incidence of 85%. Aspergillus alone is isolated in up to 45% of recipients and may be associated with bronchial anastomotic complications. The spectrum of disease ranges from asymptomatic colonization to invasive disease and systemic fungal sepsis. Invasive aspergillosis carries a mortality of 75%.

Protozoal infections

Mortality from *Pneumocystis jirovecci* (PCP) was previously significant but with the introduction of lifelong co-trimoxazole prophylaxis the incidence of infection has dramatically decreased.

10.4 Immunosuppressive medication

The majority of lung transplant recipients will receive lifelong immunosuppression using a triple-drug regime consisting of:

1. calcineurin inhibitor (ciclosporin or tacrolimus)
2. cell-cycle inhibitor (azathioprine or mycophenolate mofetil)
3. corticosteroids (prednisolone).

Important side effects include increased susceptibility to infection and calcineurin-related nephrotoxicity. Renal function needs to be carefully monitored and a degree of renal impairment is common post transplantation. Care must be taken when prescribing additional medications especially antibiotics and anti-fungal medications due to possible interactions. Therefore, all medication should be checked for potential interactions before initiation.

10.5 Assessment of transplant recipient outside the transplant centre

Lung transplant recipients with CF may present with new symptoms to either their local district hospital or their CF centre, particularly if they live a significant distance from their transplant centre. It is important to remember that not all presentations will be related to their previous transplant and that ordinary illnesses and conditions occur in the transplanted patient. However their status as a lung transplant recipient should always influence their management even for common conditions.

Table 10.1 Early complications of lung transplantation	
Anastomotic complications	• Dehiscence • Stricture • Granulation tissue obstruction.
Phrenic nerve damage	• Raised hemidiaphragm.
Pulmonary venous thrombosis	
Primary graft dysfunction	
Venous thromboembolism	
Acute rejection	
Pulmonary infection	• Bacterial • Viral • Fungal • Protozoal.
Non pulmonary infection	• Mediastinitis • Pleural collections.
Gastrointestinal	• DIOS • Peptic ulceration • GORD • Pseudomembraneous colitis.
CNS	• Ciclosporin related seizures • Multifocal leucoencephalopathy.
Metabolic	• Hypo/hyperkalaemia • Hyponatraemia • Hypomagnaeseamia • Hypocalaemia • Hypophospataemia.

Table 10.2 Late complications of lung transplant	
Airway complications	• Tracheo-bronchomalacia • Bronchial fistulae.
Malignancy	• Skin • PTLD.
Chronic allograft rejection	• Obliterative bronchiolitis.
Infection	• Bacterial • Viral • Fungal • Protozoal.
Diabetes mellitus	
Hypertension	
Dyslipidaemia	
Renal impairment	• Calcineurin inhibitor-related nephrotoxicity.

Potential causes of acute illness can be categorized as:

1. Transplant specific complications
   * acute rejection
   * rapid bronchiolitis obliterans syndrome
   * PTLD
   * opportunistic infections, etc.
2. CF specific complications
   * CF related liver disease
   * CF related diabetes
   * DIOS, etc.
3. General medical and surgical conditions
   * pulmonary embolus
   * pneumonia
   * appendicitis, etc.

The initial approach to the sick transplant patient is the same as any other patient except that special care should be taken before drug administration to consider potential interactions with immunosuppressive medication.

Patient condition and onset of deterioration determines the place of care and timing of further investigations. Basic resuscitation of the critically ill patient is the same in the lung transplant recipient. Full history and examination needs to be undertaken as standard.

10.5.1 **Fall in lung function**

If a minor fall in lung function is associated with clinical evidence of respiratory infection, then spirometry should be repeated to ensure it has normalized after treatment.

If symptoms persist, lung function fails to normalize, or there is no clinical evidence of infection then further investigations are required.

Bronchoscopy to examine the bronchial anastamoses for strictures and bronchoalveolar lavage for culture is indicated. In addition transbronchial biopsies are required to look for acute rejection.

Other than in exceptional circumstances, post-transplant bronchoscopy is best performed in the lung transplant centre where experienced transplant pathologists are available to report on transbronchial biopsies.

10.5.2 **Abnormal chest x-ray**

The chest x-ray appearance in a lung transplant recipient should always be checked against previous imaging as there may be chronic changes after transplant surgery.

If new infiltrates, nodules or effusions are identified they will require further investigation. These changes are non-specific and may represent rejection, infection or post-transplant lymphoproliferative disease. A CT scan may help to characterize the abnormalities more clearly but invariably bronchoscopic investigations as above will be required.

If a nodule cannot be characterized by bronchsocopy or imaging then a more invasive approach to biopsy will be required. Early discussion with the transplant centre should occur to help guide investigations or to transfer back for further evaluation.

10.5.3 Investigations for new onset breathlessness

- Chest x-ray
- Spirometry
- Flow volume loop if available and possible.
- Arterial blood gases if the oxygen saturations are low
- Sputum culture +/– nasopharyngeal lavage for viruses.

10.5.4 Suspected infection

If infective symptoms are present blood cultures and a full septic screen are required as source of sepsis may be outside the lungs. Any culture samples need a full work-up for an immunocompromised host—this will need to be requested specifically from local microbiology laboratories.

Targeted antibiotics, if required, are preferable to broad spectrum in lung transplant recipients but clinical judgement will dictate as to whether antibiotics are required immediately. Neutropenia is not normally present in patients on immunosuppression and therefore recipients should not automatically receive neutropenic antibiotic regimens if they present with features of infection.

The patient's lung transplant centre should be involved early for advice regarding management and antibiotics regimens. Prescription of the macrolide antibiotics, erythromycin, and clarithromycin, are contra-indicated in patients on calcineurin inhibitors due to the risk of nephrotoxicity.

References

Corris P.A. (2008) Lung transplantation for CF. *Cur. Opin. Organ Transplan.* **13**(5): 484–8.

Czebe K., Antus B., Csiszer E., Horvath I. (2006) Pulmonary infections in lung transplant recipients. *Euro. Resp. Dis.* **11**: 674–80.

Hadjiliadis D. (2007) Special considerations for patients with CF undergoing lung transplantation. *Chest* **131**: 1224–31.

International Society of Heart and Lung Transplantation. www.ishlt.org.

Levy R.D., Estenne M., Weder W., Cosio M.G. (Eds) The European Respiratory Monograph Series 'Lung Transplantation'. *European Respiratory Journal*.

Liou T.G., Woo M.S., Cahill B.C. (2006) Lung transplantation for CF. *Curr. Opin. Pul. Med.* **12**: 459–63.

Lyu D.M., Zamora M.R. (2009) Medical complications of lung transplantation. *Proc. Am. Thorac. Soc.* **6**: 101–7.

Chapter 11

Fertility, contraception and pregnancy

Frank Edenborough

Key points

Males

- Most likely to be infertile – counsel early and do a sperm test at around 18yrs
- Fatherhood is possible using sperm retrieval and in vitro fertilization (MESA and ICSI).

Females

- Menarche is likely to be delayed but regular menses is the norm unless in poor health
- All women of reproductive age should be considered fertile and offered contraception
- True fertility is unknown, but up to 2/3 women wishing to become pregnant do so naturally
- The outcome for the mother is highly dependent on her pre-conceptual health, notably weight and lung function
- For those unable to conceive, bypassing the cervical mucus plug (intrauterine insemination) or more formal in vitro fertilization techniques are available.

Pregnancy

- The outcome of pregnancy for the child is excellent
- Maintaining the mothers health with full usual CF treatment far outweighs the risk to the baby from potential fetal drug toxicity
- Risk of the child having CF depends on the partner's carrier status
- The fetus can be tested by chorionic villus sampling or amniocentesis, or in IVF a healthy embryo can be selected by pre-implantation genetic diagnosis.

11.1 General introduction

Over half the UK CF population are over 16 and likely to be taking an active interest in sexual and reproductive health. Evidence suggests high proportions are in long-term relationships and many already have children. However, many young adults are poorly educated regarding their reproductive potential and contraception is often poorly understood. Whilst accidental pregnancy occurs, and may be disastrous in CF, subfertility is an issue for many others, especially men wishing to father their own children.

11.2 Growth and puberty

Historically people with CF were on average shorter and lighter than non CF. This was assumed to be due to poor nutrition, however it remains true today despite optimum nutrition. CFTR has been found in the hypothalamus and elsewhere in the brain suggesting it may also have a role in central hormonal control. However the hypothalamic-pituitary-gonadal axis produces normal hormone levels and though puberty in men and women is delayed by up to 2 years, secondary sexual characteristics are normal. Ill health results in reduced levels of insulin and insulin like growth factors (IgF1, IgF-BP3), which have some gonadotrophin-like properties. Growth and puberty are significantly impaired in those with CF related diabetes (CFRD).

11.2.1 The effect of CFTR on reproductive tissues

Males

CFTR is found in the epididymis, vas deferens, seminal vesicles and ejaculatory ducts from as early as 18 weeks in utero. In CF, these structures are usually obstructed, atretic or absent at birth.

- 98% of men will have obstructive azoospermia and be infertile
- Congenital bilateral absence of the vas deferens (CBAVD) is seen even in mild forms of CF suggesting these structures are particularly sensitive to CFTR dysfunction
- Many infertile men with CBAVD (responsible for ~1% of male infertility) may have at least one CF mutation or indeed have subclinical CF themselves.

Females

The cervix, endometrium and fallopian tubes all express CFTR but are anatomically normal.

- Cervical goblet cell hyperplasia may lead to obstruction of the cervical os by a mucus plug resulting in subfertility
- The ovaries and breast tissues are unaffected by CFTR.

The female cycle

Menarche is on average delayed by up to 2 years (mean age ~14yrs). Primary amenorrhoea (no periods at age 16yrs) is rare but irregular cycles, anovulatory cycles with follicular cysts and secondary amenorrhoea are commonly associated with episodes of ill health and may be temporary.

11.3 Sexual development and contraception

11.3.1 Sexual function and fertility

Males

Men with CF have normal sex hormone levels, normal virilization and normal libido but some are upset reading about infertility due to confusion with impotence. Whilst 98% are likely to be infertile, potency is not affected (though some notice the ejaculate is viscid and of small volume) and it is generally felt that information on infertility, with clarification that sexual function is normal, should be given during transition to adult services.

- Azoospermia should be checked for after age 18 (because there are no normative values for younger men) during periods of good health and after sexual abstinence for 3–4 days.

Females

Coitarche in women with CF is at the same age as in non-CF. Sexual function is normal although vaginal dryness and thrush (associated with antibiotics and diabetes) is more common and may be associated with dyspareunia.

- The potential fertility of women with CF is unknown as many choose not to have children but studies report success rates of around 2/3 of women wishing to conceive doing so without recourse to assisted reproductive techniques.

11.3.2 Contraception

Success rates with correct use given in brackets.

Males

- Men should not assume they are infertile until they have had a sperm test
- All men with CF should use a condom (98%) for all casual sexual encounters to prevent sexually transmitted diseases.

Females

- The range of contraceptive choices for women with CF is as for non-CF women
- Only condoms (98%), and the femidom (95%), protect against sexually transmitted diseases.

1. Barrier contraceptives
- The cap or diaphragm (92–96%) should be used in conjunction with spermicidal cream.

2. Oral contraceptives (98%)
- Combined oestrogen/progestogen containing pills (cyclical, permitting menses) should contain at least 30mcg oestrogen
- Progesterone only pills prevent menstruation, may be complicated by break-through bleeding and may potentiate osteopoenia.

Potential complications

There is a theoretical risk of reduced absorption during new antibiotic courses. Barrier precautions are recommended during and for 7 days after antibiotic treatment. Increased sputum viscosity, reduced lung function, impaired liver function and glycaemic control, and thrombogenesis in the context of implantable venous access devices are all theoretical risks and should be monitored for at least the first 6 months.

3. Injectable contraceptives (>99%).
- Long acting progestogens can be given IM (e.g. Depo-Provera®) or as implanted rods (Implanon®) in those for whom the pill is unsuitable. Both may be associated with break-through bleeding and osteopenia. Implanon may be more suitable for long-term use with less osteopenia and quicker return of ovulation on removal.

4. Intrauterine devices (IUDs) (98–99%).
- May contain copper or elute progesterone and should be discussed with and inserted by a specialist.

5. Tubal ligation.
- This may be considered in someone decidedly against having a child, someone with a child who wishes no more, or in someone too ill to consider a future pregnancy who is struggling with other contraceptive means.

Key Point

Pregnancy has been reported in severely underweight CF women on transplant lists. Outcomes are usually bad for the mother whether the pregnancy is completed or termination is performed. All women with CF should be considered fertile and adequate contraception offered.

11.4 Reproductive genetics and counselling

- CF is an autosomal recessive state and all gametes will have an abnormal CF gene, i.e. all offspring will be (at least) carriers
- The risk of someone with CF having a CF child is entirely dependent upon the partner. If the partner is a carrier, the risk is 1:2, if untested (based on European carrier frequency of 1:25) the risk is 1:50, and if tested and not a carrier the risk is around 1:700.

11.4.1 Genetic counselling

Ideally discussions with the couple should start well before conception. The nature of the disease (CF), the unaffected carrier status and whether wider family members should be informed if a gene is identified in the partner should be discussed. The specific risks of vertical transmission, implications of potential subfertility, the potential effect of CF drugs and treatment on the pregnancy and potential child, and the effect of pregnancy on a woman with CF should be explored.

11.4.2 Psychological counselling

People with CF generally wish to be normal and many will wish to have a family. Some girls, whether in a relationship or not, express a desire to leave something of themselves behind. Sub/infertility may be devastating to a person with CF wishing to have a child. Perhaps worse is when a woman is advised she should not become pregnant because she is too unwell to either conceive or carry a pregnancy, or when an accidentally pregnant woman with advanced CF is told that a therapeutic termination may be the only way to save her.

- Couples should be advised that there is a real possibility the partner with CF will not survive long enough to see their child reach adulthood and may be too sick to participate in childcare
- Many multidisciplinary CF teams have psychologists within them who are best placed to explore these issues.

11.5 Assisted conception

11.5.1 Assisted conception techniques
Males

Although the ejaculate is azoospermic, men with CF do produce normal sperm, which can be retrieved from the testes and used with artificial reproductive techniques. PESA (percutaneous epididymal sperm aspiration), TESA and TESE (testicular sperm aspiration/extraction, by biopsy) can yield sufficient sperm of good quality even in ill health to facilitate pregnancy by intracytoplasmic sperm injection (ICSI).

> **Box 11.1 *In vitro* fertilization**
>
> Assuming a woman is otherwise reasonably well from her CF, IVF is usually considered if baseline tests are normal (including hormone profile, pelvic and transvaginal ultrasound). Superovulation is induced and developing follicles are monitored by ultrasound and oestradiol levels. Ova are 'ripened' with human chorionic gonadotrophin (HCG) and harvested 34–38hrs later by transvaginal follicular aspiration under sedation. Fertilization is achieved by incubation with washed sperm for 48–72hrs or by ICSI. Embryo transfer by intrauterine injection occurs at the 6–8 cell stage on day 2 or 3 post fertilization. Success rates of up to 33% per cycle can be expected. Success rates decline after maternal age 30.

To optimize the chance of a pregnancy the (healthy) partner of a man with CF will have to undergo investigation and treatment similar to those of a CF woman trying to conceive – see below.

Females

In healthy women with CF who cannot conceive the most likely cause is the cervical mucus plug which can be by-passed by intrauterine sperm injection. However many women less well with CF will have difficulty conceiving and require full investigation and undergo in vitro fertilization techniques (IVF).

- Pregnancy is unlikely in the very underweight (BMI<18kg/m^2) or in those with secondary amenorrhoea due to significant pulmonary or hepatic disease. These women are unlikely to be considered for IVF.

11.5.2 Genetic testing of the fetus

When a woman with CF presents already pregnant and the father's genotype cannot be tested, or he is a carrier of an identifiable gene, chorionic villus sampling (8–12 weeks) or amniocentesis (12–18 weeks) can be performed to test to see whether the fetus has CF. These techniques were also offered to couples pregnant through IVF but nowadays with pre-implantation genetic diagnosis (PGD) it is possible to take cells from the developing embryo (day 2–3) and test for CF. Couples may choose to have only a healthy (carrier) embryo implanted, avoiding the risk of miscarriage with CVS (1–2%) or amniocentesis (1%).

Current CF genotype testing techniques are limited, and do not reduce the risk of a CF child to zero as some genes cannot be routinely identified prior to conception or with CVS/amniocentesis.

11.6 Pregnancy in women with CF

11.6.1 Background

The first pregnancy in a woman with CF was reported in 1960. Subsequent cases and annual reports from the North American CF Database confirmed pregnancy was increasingly common. Early reviews suggested pregnancy was only likely to succeed in healthy women with CF (late diagnosis, pancreatic sufficient, good weight and lung function, no diabetes). Increasingly pregnancy is seen in pancreatic insufficient women and there are numerous reports of women surviving pregnancy despite impaired lung function.

- In general, healthy women can expect a normal pregnancy aiming for normal vaginal delivery at term with the opportunity to breast feed the infant thereafter
- In those less well, poor weight, or weight gain in pregnancy, and poor lung function predict the likelihood of increased respiratory exacerbations, increased hospital visits, intensification of treatment, a propensity to premature delivery (due to maternal concerns) via assisted delivery whether planned or as an emergency.

Key Point

Whilst some women report their best ever health in pregnancy, even healthy women may experience a faster than expected decline in their CF health and may not fully recover after delivery.

11.6.2 Preparing for pregnancy

Counselling

Risk of pregnancy. Is it right for her? Who will care for child or for her if she is ill? Survival with child, and fitting treatment around childcare.

Genetic counselling

Get the partner tested. If he is a carrier, risk of CF is 50:50; how do they feel about a child with CF or would they try to avoid it or terminate a pregnancy? If he is not a carrier the child will be a carrier but risk of CF is minimal (around 1:700 if common mutations excluded).

Optimize medication

Continue all routine CF medication. Avoid starting new medication periconception. Recommend full treatment of any chest infection before contraception stops. (NB no evidence of teratogenicity of any CF therapies to date)

- Start folic acid 400mcg and continue to 14 weeks
- Check vitamin A levels and continue usual supplemental dose unless high/low levels (both associated with teratogenicity)
- Check iron and consider supplementation if low.

Optimize nutrition

Aim for preconception body weight, >90% ideal

- Plan for 300+kcal extra a day (up to 150% Recommended Daily Requirements, RDR)
- Consider energy dense foods, oral supplements or early instigation of NG feeding or PEG (difficult to do in late pregnancy).
- Aim for weight gain of at least 10kg during pregnancy (more if underweight).

Physiotherapy

Optimize airway clearance and review adherence, sequence, technique and necessity of inhaled medication and exercise regimes

- Breathlessness in the first trimester is hormonally driven and women should be advised this is likely
- In late pregnancy the expanding uterus compresses basal areas of the lungs increasing the risk of sputum trapping and infection
- Unlike non-CF pregnancies there is frequently a decline in FEV_1 and FVC as pregnancy progresses
- General cardiovascular fitness, core stability and strength is important
- Pelvic floor exercises should be encouraged. Cough urinary incontinence is common in girls with CF and is likely to get worse during and after pregnancy.

11.6.3 Monitoring during pregnancy

Lung function, weight and glucose homeostasis should be monitored carefully throughout pregnancy.

- Women should probably be seen at least 2 monthly until ~32 weeks, then monthly until 38 weeks and weekly thereafter (remember to try and coincide/liaise with obstetric visits)
- Blood sugar should be measured on each visit, especially with exacerbations
- Oral glucose tolerance tests, routinely done in pregnancy at 20 weeks, should be performed at onset of pregnancy, at 20 weeks and at end of 2nd trimester, or if there is any doubt.

11.6.4 Management of CF during pregnancy

Respiratory exacerbation and declining lung function with hypoxia pose the greatest threat to mother and hence to baby. Any decline should be treated aggressively with review of airway clearance, bronchodilators, oral antibiotics and a low threshold for intravenous antibiotics, and with supplemental oxygen if SpO_2 falls below 95%.

- Conventional dual antibiotic therapy with a beta lactam and aminoglycoside (with close monitoring of levels) is safe. There are no reports of fetal ototoxicty in mothers treated with these regimens and the risk to the baby from hypoxia or sepsis far outweighs the potential risk from drug therapy
- Poor weight gain should be investigated by reviewing actual calorie/nutrient intake, enzyme usage, and use of supplemental feeding as required
- Be vigilant for pregnancy related hyperemesis gravidarum, reflux and dyspepsia, and constipation (or worsening CF related distal obstruction symptoms)
- The onset of gestational diabetes should be treated with maintained high calorie intake covered by insulin.

11.6.5 Obstetric considerations in CF pregnancy

As soon as pregnancy is confirmed, close liaison must begin between the obstetric and CF teams. This includes between the CF specialist nurse and midwives, and between the CF physician, the obstetrician, and an anaesthetist familiar with high-risk obstetric cases. Visits should coincide to reduce inconvenience to the mother and avoid duplication of tests.

- The incidence of obstetric complications is not increased in CF. Occasional bleeding, hypertension, and similar rates of tubal pregnancy and miscarriage to the non-CF population have been reported
- Most problems encountered will have an origin in the mother's CF health, namely poor maternal weight gain and intrauterine growth retardation (not a feature of CF per se)
- Early discussion with the mother must consider preferred analgesia and mode of delivery, but must also cover the possibility of planned or emergency early intervention and delivery if either mother or baby is in crisis.

Analgesia

Epidural anaesthesia early in stage 1 of delivery gives good analgesia, saves energy for stage 2 (delivery), and facilitates natural childbirth but can be converted to spinal anaesthesia for instrumentation or caesarean section if required. It can also be left in situ to allow early mobilization and chest physiotherapy after delivery.

Mode and timing of delivery

Whilst normal vaginal delivery at term is the outcome of choice, some women may choose caesarean section and others may be too unwell to manage natural childbirth without assistance. The obstetrician and physician may plan for early induction at or before 40 weeks where the mother is struggling, if the baby is big (macrosomia with diabetes) or the mother is small (due to CF). In advanced CF, or in the context of severe decline during pregnancy, steroids may be given to prepare the fetal lungs with planned delivery any time after 32 weeks, or in the eventuality of an emergency delivery.

11.6.6 Breast feeding

'Breast is best' (for the baby), even in CF, since breast milk composition is essentially normal. Breast feeding however requires up to an additional 500kcal day and may be hard for a CF mother to sustain. Formula feed supplementation may be necessary but breast feeding should be encouraged for at least 3 weeks.

11.6.7 Pregnancy after transplantation

- Many women who undergo successful lung transplantation see it as a second chance and consider the opportunity to have a child. Many successful pregnancies have been reported in solid organ transplants including kidney, liver and heart. However there is less experience of pregnancy after heart lung or double lung transplant
- Successful pregnancies have been reported but there is a high incidence of eclampsia, prematurity and graft rejection
- Pregnancy seems to exacerbate rejection (despite up-titrating of therapy to account for increased volume of distribution)
- General advice remains cautious.

> **Key Point**
>
> Pregnancy is not recommended within 2 years of transplantation, or if there have been significant episodes of rejection or declining lung function since transplant.

11.6.8 Fetal outcome in CF pregnancy

Early studies suggested increased perinatal mortality but this is no longer the case due to advances in obstetric and paediatric care and special care baby units.

- Fetal anomalies have been reported in CF pregnancies but none have been attributed to either CF, its treatment or transplant related treatment
- No long-term studies have been performed on babies to CF parents and the potential for physical or psychological sequelae as a consequence of having a sick parent, or of losing a parent during childhood, remain unknown.

11.6.9 Maternal outcomes in CF pregnancy

Since early reports appeared in the literature, it has been clear that some women with CF do badly during pregnancy, experiencing catastrophic change in lung function and weight that is not recovered in the post partum years. Maternal survival with child is often poor. What is not clear is whether these women were likely to do badly even if they were not pregnant. The markers of poor outcome for pregnancy in CF are the same as for poor outcome for CF generally. The literature on the effect of pregnancy on survival in women with CF compared to women who do not get pregnant is dominated by the only large and adequately statistically powered study from the North American database.

- Women who become pregnant were healthier than those who did not. Women who became pregnant had better survival overall
- When the data were corrected for disease severity, even women with FEV1 <40% appeared to do better than equivalent non pregnant controls
- The group most at risk was those women who conceived very young (<18).

> **Key Point**
>
> 20% of mothers will die before their child's 10th birthday, and if FEV_1<40%, 40% will die before child's 10th birthday.

11.6.10 Contraindications to pregnancy

The only absolute contraindications remain pulmonary hypertension and cor pulmonale. Relative contraindications are FEV_1<60%, BMI<18, CF related diabetes and infection with *B. cenocepacia*.

11.6.11 Termination of pregnancy in CF

Termination of pregnancy may be requested for accidental pregnancy for psychosocial reasons or may be necessitated by poor maternal health or for obstetric reasons, e.g. anomalies.

- Medical termination using oral mifepristone followed by prostaglandin vaginally or by mouth avoids the need for anaesthesia and instrumentation
- Surgical termination may be necessary as determined by the obstetrician.

References

Edenborough F.P. (2001) Respiratory Diseases in Pregnancy 4. Women with cystic fibrosis and their potential for reproduction. *Thorax* **56**: 649–55.

Edenborough F.P., Borgo G., Knoop C., *et al.* (2008) Guidelines for the management of pregnancy in women with cystic fibrosis. *J. Cyst. Fibros.* **7**: S2–32.

Goss C.H (2003) The effect of pregnancy on survival in women with Cystic Fibrosis. *Chest* **124**: 1460–8.

Gyi K.M. (2006) Pregnancy in cystic fibrosis lung transplant recipients: Case series and review. *J. Cyst. Fibros.* **5**: 171–6.

Chapter 12

Future treatments

Uta Griesenbach, Jane Davies and
Eric Alton

> **Key points**
> - Increased understanding of CF pathophysiology is leading to new therapies
> - Several gene therapy trials have established proof-of-principle for gene transfer in the airways, but a gene therapy-based treatment has not yet been developed
> - Small molecule drugs directed at class-specific CFTR mutations are showing promise in early phase trials
> - Drugs aimed at restoring hydration of the airway surface have been shown to improve mucociliary clearance
> - Increasing numbers of antibiotics are being formulated for both nebulization and inhalation.

12.1 Introduction

CF is an attractive target for genetic and molecular therapies aimed at correcting the basic defect. It is a common single gene disorder with an abbreviated life expectancy, the site of major pathology (the lung) is easily accessible, and there is evidence to suggest that partial correction of the underlying defect would be able to achieve clinical benefit. We are increasingly defining the mechanisms by which defective CFTR results in clinical disease, and there are a number of points of intervention where novel therapies could effect a 'cure' (Figure 12.1). In reality, it has been much harder to circumvent the body's immune system and achieve effective gene transfer and expression. Increasingly, novel therapies are directed at alternative steps in the gene expression pathway.

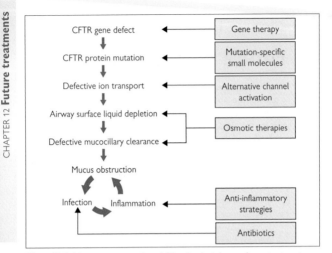

Figure 12.1 Schematic presentation of CF pathophysiology and new treatment strategies that are currently being developed for the different aspects of disease aetiology.

12.2 **Gene therapy**

CF has been at the forefront of gene therapy research. Since cloning of the CFTR gene in 1989, 25 phase I/II clinical trials, involving approximately 420 CF patients, have been carried out using a variety of viral and non-viral gene transfer agents (GTAs). Although many of these trials established proof-of-principle for gene transfer in the airways, a gene therapy-based treatment has not yet been developed. Not surprisingly airway epithelial cells, which have evolved to keep foreign particles out of the lung, are difficult to transfect. The GTAs employed so far can be divided into those derived at least in part from viruses that typically infect the airway epithelium, and artificial liposome vectors, containing a copy of the CFTR gene. Viral vectors are typically highly effective at infecting and transfecting airway cells, but induce an immune response that limits repeat administration, and only some are capable of carrying the large CFTR gene. Artificial liposomal vectors on the other hand are designed to be administered repeatedly, but suffer from lower rates of transfection. Each of the two approaches has both merits and significant remaining challenges.

12.2.1 **Clinical studies**

Viral vectors

Despite encouraging results in nasal and pulmonary tissues of pre-clinical models, and despite being well-tolerated at low to intermediate doses in humans, adenovirus-mediated gene transfer in the absence of epithelial damage has been inefficient in CF patients. This is mainly due to the absence of the coxsackie-adenovirus receptor on the apical surface of the majority of human airway epithelial cells, and highlights the important differences in receptor distribution between animal models and man.

Adenoviruses were superseded by first generation adeno-associated viruses (AAV). Several clinical trials have been carried out in the nose, sinus and lungs of CF patients all demonstrating that one of these, AAV2, is safe even when repeatedly administered. However, a more recent phase II trial assessing efficacy of repeated administration (three doses one month apart) failed to significantly improve lung function and has been discontinued.

The use of viral vectors for chronic diseases such as CF is currently limited by effective cellular and humoral immune responses against the virus, which prevent re-administration of the vectors. Suitable strategies that prevent immune responses and are compatible with use in CF patients have so far not been identified.

Non-viral vectors

Nine clinical trials have evaluated non-viral gene transfer to nasal or lung epithelium. The majority of these studies have shown approximately 25% correction of the chloride transport defect in either the nasal or pulmonary epithelium (Figure 12.2). In contrast to viral GTAs, non-viral formulations are more likely to be able to be administered repeatedly, and proof-of-principle for this has been demonstrated in man. Despite these promising studies it is not known if non-viral gene transfer agents, which are less efficient than viral vectors, will be able to correct clinically relevant endpoints such as infection and inflammation in the CF lung. The UK CF Gene Therapy Consortium (http://www.cfgenetherapy.org.uk) has identified the most efficient non-viral GTA currently available for airway transfection and will, over the next few years, assess whether repeated administration of this complex can alter clinically relevant endpoints in CF.

12.2.2 **Pre-clinical developments**

Viral vectors

Helper-dependent ('gutted') adenoviral vectors, which are depleted of all viral genes, have been developed, but do not currently prevent induction of immune responses. Research into the optimal AAV-vectors

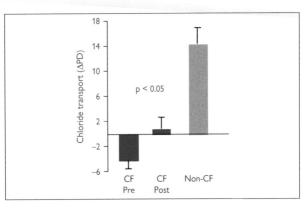

Figure 12.2 Partial correction of low chloride transport in lungs of CF patients after administration of a CFTR plasmid complexed with cationic lipid. "Pre" = chloride transport in CF lung before gene therapy, "Post" = chloride transport in CF lung after gene therapy, "Non-CF" = chloride transport in non-CF lung. Data shown are mean±SEM. Adapted from Alton E, et. al. (1999) *Lancet* **353**: 947–54, with permission from Elsevier.

for airway transduction is being pursued actively. Various natural isoforms have been identified and assessed for airway transfection. In addition, molecular evolution techniques are currently utilized to generate novel AAV vectors. Strategies to overcome the AAV packaging problem, thereby allowing incorporation of stronger promoters in addition to the large CFTR gene, are being assessed. However, the feasibility of repeated AAV administration is still unresolved. Results have varied greatly, and may depend on the host, delivery route and AAV serotype tested.

Most recently, lentiviral vectors, which integrate into the genome of the target cell, have been developed for airway gene transfer. Gene expression *in vivo* persists in mouse airway epithelium for the lifetime of the animal. Importantly, lentiviruses can be repeatedly administered to the airways of mice, although it is currently unclear how the virus evades the immune system.

Non-viral vectors

Over the last few years there have not been many convincing advances in improving non-viral gene vectors for the airway gene transfer. However, improvements in the plasmids used for non-viral gene transfer are at least as important as improving the lipid or polymer vector. A good example is the generation of plasmids completely devoid of pro-inflammatory unmethylated 'CpG' sequences in the bacterial DNA. This has reduced inflammatory responses and prolonged gene expression in mouse models. The optimal combination of non-viral vector and plasmid DNA will ultimately determine efficiency and safety.

12.3 **Mutation specific therapies**

The classes of mutations and effect they have on protein production/ function have been discussed in Chapter 1 and are illustrated in Figure 1.2. Based on an increased understanding in this area, several novel approaches to therapy have been devised, some of which have reached the stage of clinical trials.

12.3.1 **Class I mutations**

These premature truncation (stop) mutations result in an absence of full-length CFTR protein. The initial observation that certain members of the aminoglycoside family could facilitate read-through of these mutations and subsequent translation of full-length protein, has led to synthetic drugs with similar properties being trialled. Such drugs do not affect the normal termination of translation in non-mutated genes as the normal DNA 'stop' sequences are flanked both upstream and downstream by specific enhancing sequences.

Of the newly discovered molecules, PTC124 has been shown partially to restore chloride secretion on nasal potential difference testing. Certain class I mutations may be more amenable to this type of correction than others and multi-centre phase III studies are currently underway to determine how these changes correlate with improvements in clinical status.

12.3.2 **Class II mutations**

The commonest cause worldwide of CF is a mutation in this class: Phe508del. Full length protein is produced but is mis-folded and therefore incorrectly processed: instead of trafficking to the apical cell surface it undergoes degradation. Early experiments confirmed that incubation at reduced temperature encouraged trafficking, after which Phe508del protein was able to function as a chloride channel, albeit at reduced levels of efficiency. Subsequent work has revealed increased rates of turnover at the apical cell membrane in addition to this trafficking problem.

The concept of certain molecules facilitating trafficking has led to the terms 'molecular chaperoning' and a search for co-called 'corrector' drugs. 4-phenylbutyrate has been demonstrated to increase CFTR function, although whether this is via inhibition of the natural degradation process, or an increase in CFTR expression is unclear. Early clinical trials of this agent provided proof-of-principle on the basis of changes in nasal potential difference, although clinical development has been limited by side effects.

Miglustat, an alpha glucosidase inhibitor, in clinical use for the inherited metabolic disorder Gaucher's disease, has been shown to restore chloride secretion in both cultured CF cells and CF mice. Results from a recent Phase II clinical trial are awaited.

High throughput screening has led several groups to identify potentially promising small molecule approaches; one such drug, VX809, is currently in clinical trial.

12.3.3 **Class III mutations**

These mutations result in full length protein which reaches its correct position on the apical cell surface but which fails to respond to activation by cAMP-mediated phosphorylation. These so-called 'gating' mutations therefore lead to a reduced chloride transport activity of the CFTR protein. Encouraging results have been reported for VX770, a member of the 'potentiator' class of drugs which increases chloride transport of the CFTR. In placebo controlled trials, VX770 has been shown to correct sweat chloride values into the non-CF range and to significantly improve chloride secretion, when assessed by nasal potential difference. Larger phase III clinical trials are currently being initiated to explore the clinical benefits associated with such electrophysiological changes.

12.4 **Other agents**

12.4.1 **Alternative ion channels**

Denufosol is a P2Y2 receptor agonist that increases chloride secretion through non-CFTR channels by increasing intracellular calcium concentrations. Early phase trials demonstrated improvements in nasal potential difference and mucociliary clearance and later small, but statistically significant, increases in lung function were reported. Multi-centre trials are underway.

12.4.2 **Osmotic therapies**

Mannitol is a non-absorbable osmotic sugar, which was shown in early phase studies to improve both mucociliary and cough clearance in patients with CF. It improved FEV_1 over a short period of 2 weeks, and a phase III trial has recently been completed demonstrating improvements in FEV_1 and frequency of pulmonary exacerbations over a 6 month period. Theoretical concerns of an increase in bacterial growth related to the nutritional functions of the compound appear to be unfounded.

12.5 **New antimicrobial therapies**

Although there are many antibacterial agents available for systemic use, there is a relative paucity of relevant drugs for topical use. Aztreonam has now been formulated for nebulization and in a series of well-conducted clinical trials has resulted in improvements in lung function compared to placebo; head-to-head trials are currently underway comparing aztreonam with nebulized tobramycin solution (TOBI®).

A liposomal formulation of the aminoglycoside amikacin has been developed for nebulisation, with promising initial results and trials of inhaled ciprofloxacin are also planned. Both colistin and tobramycin have been formulated as dry powders with an emphasis on rapid, easy delivery having the potential to improve quality of life.

Trial data confirming non-inferiority to licensed nebulized drugs is likely to be required before these drugs will be granted marketing authorization.

Trials of anti-pseudomonal vaccine approaches have, to date, been disappointing (see Chapter 3). An increased understanding of mechanisms of infection, such as quorum sensing and biofilms and the recognition, with molecular tools, that many more organisms exist within the CF lower airway than has been thought, may lead to new antimicrobial approaches in the future.

12.6 **Assessing new treatments**

The design of clinical trials in CF is becoming more complex and challenging. Whereas several decades ago, patients deteriorated rapidly and had a short life expectancy, predicted survival of today's children is around 40 years and many live relatively healthy lives, albeit at the cost of time spent on multiple treatments. This means that certain previously appropriate outcome measures (rate of decline in lung function and mortality) are now inappropriate for the vast majority of trials, and that more sophisticated surrogate measures have to be designed and applied.

Which of these surrogates are chosen, ranging from basic molecular assays to standard clinical measurements, will depend in part on the intervention being applied, on the severity of the group being studied, and the time period available over which change can be measured. Levels of CFTR transgene mRNA are limited in applicability to gene therapy trials, whereas antibody-based techniques to detect apically-localized CFTR would be useful in this context and also with small molecule drugs aimed directly at certain classes of CFTR mutation (e.g. premature stop mutations).

CFTR function is often assessed electrophysiologically using an *in vivo* technique, epithelial potential difference. Baseline measurements largely reflect sodium absorption and application of zero chloride solutions and isoprenaline (which stimulates cAMP) allows a highly sensitive assessment of chloride transport; this is the primary outcome measure in many of the trials outlined above. Alternatively, for systemically applied drugs, sweat electrolyte measurements provide a simple, non-invasive end-point assay.

Several strategies aimed at improving hydration of the airway surface have been assessed with mucociliary clearance scans, where clearance of inhaled labelled particles is followed over time. For larger, later phase studies, relevant outcome measures might include bacterial load, inflammatory markers (sputum, exhaled breath, blood, bronchoalveolar lavage), lung function testing (both conventional methods and more novel techniques such as the multiple breath washout), reduction in the frequency of exacerbations and CT scans. The choice of which of these measures to employ will depend crucially on the intervention being applied, the sensitivity of the assay to detect change and the phase of study.

12.7 **Conclusions**

Considerable progress in the development of new therapies based around the basic CF defect has been made in the two decades following cloning of the CF gene. Importantly, these therapies are aimed at multiple targets along the pathophysiological pathway, thereby spreading the risk of failure. Academics, charities and industry have combined in unique partnerships to address issues related to a clear unmet need but in the context of a relatively small patient population. There is considerable optimism, but this needs to be balanced by the recognition that no treatment aimed at the basic defect is yet in routine clinical use.

References

Alton E.W., Stern M., Farley R., *et al.* (1999) Cationic lipid-mediated CFTR gene transfer to the lungs and nose of patients with cystic fibrosis: a double-blind placebo-controlled trial. *Lancet* **353**: 947–54.

Boucher R.C. (2007) Airway surface dehydration in cystic fibrosis: pathogenesis and therapy. *Annu. Rev. Med.* **58**: 157–70.

Davies J.C., Alton E.W. (2009) Monitoring respiratory disease severity in cystic fibrosis. *Respir. Care* **54**: 606–17.

Dudley M.N., Loutit J., Griffith D.C. (2008) Aerosol antibiotics: considerations in pharmacological and clinical evaluation. *Curr. Opin. Biotechnol.* **19**: 637–43.

Griesenbach U. and Alton E.W. (2009) Gene transfer to the lung: lessons learned from more than 2 decades of CF gene therapy. *Adv. Drug Deliv. Rev.* **61**: 128–39.

Mitomo K., Griesenbach U., Inoue M., *et al.* (2010) Toward gene therapy for cystic fibrosis using a lentivirus pseudotyped with Sendai virus envelopes. *Molecular Therapy* doi:10.1038/mt.2010.13

Sinn P.L., Arias A.C., Brogden K.A., McCray P.B. Jr. (2008) Lentivirus vector can be readministered to nasal epithelia without blocking immune responses. *J. Virol.* **82**: 10684–92.

Zeitlin P.L. (2007) Emerging drug treatments for cystic fibrosis. *Expert Opin. Emerg. Drugs* **12**: 329–36.

Appendix

Useful internet resources

www.cftrust.org.uk
Website of the national UK CF charity. Contains information for patients and links to standards of care and consensus guidelines for management of CF

www.cysticfibrosismedicine.com
The Leeds method of treatment and management of CF in adults and children.

www.cochrane.org
Cochrane collaboration of systematic reviews, including a number specific to CF

www.ecfs.eu
European Cystic Fibrosis Society, with links to useful guidelines and consensus reports

www.ecorn-cf.eu
Europe-wide advice forum for patients, carers, and health professionals.

www.cfgenetherapy.org.uk
Website of the CF Trust-funded gene therapy research consortium, currently engaged in preparation for clinical trials (2010).

www.cff.org
Patient-centred web forum of the US national CF charity

www.mycysticfibrosis.com
US patient-centred website and discussion forum

Index

Page references to Boxes, Figures and Tables are in *italic* print

C